THEORY Z
Hospital Management
Lessons from Japan

Seth B. Goldsmith, Sc.D.

Professor of Public Health
Health Administration Program
University of Massachusetts
Amherst

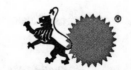

AN ASPEN PUBLICATION®

Aspen Systems Corporation
Rockville, Maryland
Royal Tunbridge Wells
1984

Library of Congress Cataloging in Publication Data

Goldsmith, Seth.
Theory Z hospital management.

"An Aspen publication."
1. Hospitals—Japan—Administration.   2. Hospitals—
United States—Administration.   I. Title.   [DNLM:
1. Hospital administration—Japan. WX 150 G624t]
RA990.J3G64   1983   362.1′1′068   83-15574
ISBN: 0-89443-949-9

Publisher: John Marozsan
Editor-in-Chief: Michael Brown
Executive Managing Editor: Margot Raphael
Editorial Services: Eileen Higgins
Printing and Manufacturing: Debbie Collins

Library of Congress Catalog Card Number: 83-15574
ISBN: 0-89443-949-9

Printed in the United States of America

1   2   3   4   5

Table of Contents

Preface   vii

Acknowledgments   xiii

PART 1—PROBLEM, PERSPECTIVE, AND POTENTIAL   1

Chapter   1—The American Hospital Dilemma   3

    Out-of-Control Health Care Costs   3
    Finding Ways To Save Money   4
    The Burden on the Hospitals   4
    Hospital Boards—Real or Imaginary Power?   7
    The Problem with Administrators   7
    Solutions   8
    Conclusions   9

Chapter   2—Management—The Japanese Way   11

    Introduction   11
    The Magic Potion of Japanese Managerial
      Success   11
    Stereotyping Japanese Industry   12
    Japan, Inc.: Does It Exist?   12
    The Japanese Labor Scene   13
    The Elements of Japanese Managerial Success   15
    Disadvantages of the Japanese System   20
    Profesional versus Group Identity   20
    Rising through the Japanese Corporation   20

75042

Implications of the Japanese System 21
Application to Hospitals 22

Chapter 3—The Japanese Health Service: An Overview 27
Naoki Ikegami and Seth B. Goldsmith

Historical Background 27
Health Insurance System 29
Problems Facing the Future 33

Chapter 4—Hospital Management in Japan:
An Overview 37

Japanese and U.S. Hospital Management Practices 37
Hospital Administration Training 38
Case Descriptions 39

PART II—CASE STUDIES AND SURVEY 45

Chapter 5—The Public Corporation Hospital 47

Introduction 47
Personnel Administration 48
Nursing Department 51
Radiology Department 54
Business Management 55
Discussion 56

Chapter 6—The Kitashinagawa Hospital 59

Dr. Minoru Kohno, Hospital Founder 59
Facilities 60
Patient Volume 61
Staffing 61
Budget 61
Information Management 62
Managerial Organization 62
Managerial Philosophy 62
Radiology Department 63
Nursing Department 64
Personnel 64
Discussion 65

Chapter   7—St. Luke's International Hospital **67**

History 67
Hospital Organization 68
Finance 69
Nursing 70
Radiology 75
Personnel 76
Discussion 81

**Chapter   8—Hospital Worker's Attitudes and Opinions in
        Japan and the United States** **85**

Introduction 85
Methodological Notes and Limitations 86
Sample Age Differences 92
Selecting a Place To Work 93
Chi-Square Analysis 97
Job Leaving Attitudes 100
Attitudes toward Hospital Administration 111
Attitudes toward Supervision 112
Opinions about the Organization 113
Summary 114

PART III—CONCLUSIONS **117**

**Chapter   9—Summary and Discussion: Japanese Hospitals
        and Management** **119**

The Japanese Hospital 119
Management of the Japanese Hospital 122
Japanese Style Management in Japanese Hospitals ... 124
The Magic Formula 128

Chapter   10—An Agenda for American Hospital Management **129**

A Five-Point Agenda for Change 130
Payoffs and Risks 134

**Appendix A—Annotated Bibliogrpahy of Hospital Administration
        Books in Japanese** **135**

Appendix B—Selected English-Language Readings on
            Health Care in Japan 139

Index 141

Preface

Everyday at noon, a 689,000-pound Boeing 747 lumbers away from the Pan Am building at Kennedy Airport, races down the runway, and begins its ascent to a cruising altitude of 39,000 feet. This 350-passenger jet will, in the course of the next 13 hours and 15 minutes, burn almost all of its 47,000 gallons of aviation fuel and in the process, lose 315,000 pounds. At a cruising speed of 550 miles per hour, the jet takes a route that first traverses New York State and Quebec Province. Then it continues across the Yukon Territory, where it seems that one can almost reach out and touch the mountain tops; over Nome, Alaska; and then south of the Aleutian Islands and Siberia. Finally it begins its final descent into Narita Airport, 66 kilometers west of Tokyo. Fourteen time zones have been crossed and, for me, the expectation is that more is different than the same.

The evening before I left for Tokyo in December 1981 was spent wrapping gifts for people I had either corresponded with or expected to meet in Japan. To be on the safe side, I brought dozens of extra gifts. They proved to be necessary.

Why was I on this trip in the first place? Sixteen years earlier I had visited Japan as a tourist, for a two-week stay. My impressions at that time were of a bustling and exciting country, blending much of the beauty and traditions of the Orient with the technology of the West. This trip was more purposeful: not a tour of the Tokyo Tower, a Nikon factory, or the Ginza, rather, a trip to learn about hospital management in Japan.

Why travel half way around the world to learn about hospital management? My reason for making this journey was largely related to the myriad problems of hospital management in the United States and my desire to see if the so-called Japanese approach to industrial management had a successful analogue in the hospital industry—an analogue that could be imported to the United States.

The problems of hospital administration often center on the rapidly escalating costs of health care. The United States, with its 7,000 hospitals, spent an estimated $322 billion in 1982 on health care—up almost 15 percent from the previous fiscal year. On a per capita basis, the expenditures for personal health services have risen from $663 in 1977 to $1,043 in 1981. These increased costs are due to a variety of factors, including those areas over which administrators have little control, such as inflation or new technological developments. But as one looks more closely at the health care expenditure data, two pieces of information become evident. First, the largest slice of health care dollars is spent in hospitals, an estimated $112 billion in 1982; and second, within hospitals, the greatest amount is spent on staffing, roughly 60 cents of every dollar. The labor intensive nature of the hospital and health care industry thus represents an opportunity for savings since administrators, through their formal authority and responsibility as well as their informal leadership, can have a crucial impact on such sensitive areas as productivity, innovation, turnover, and quality of work life.

But what we now have in American hospital administration is the following dilemma: In a time of increasingly better trained management, there are more and more management problems, many of which affect an organization's economic and spiritual viability. The operations researchers, with their staffing or patient queuing models, have come and gone. The industrial engineers, à la Frederick Winslow Taylor, with their dietary or central supply department efficiency studies, have not solved the problems. The computer models for financial management, in particular, those focusing on maximizing reimbursement, have clear value, but they are attacking the "increasing the revenue" issue not the "decreasing the cost" problem. The multiple hospital system promises us the efficiency of economies of scale; as of yet, we have mostly seen increased costs and more (and better) jobs in corporate headquarters. Perhaps there are no solutions—only partial answers.

Meanwhile the industrial sector of the U.S. economy is not immune from similar concerns. A laundry list of industrial sector problems reminds one of the hospital field: high turnover, low productivity, poor quality workmanship, and low morale. And, in the industrial sector we have also seen an explosion in high-quality management education. Indeed, the conventional wisdom is that the M.B.A. degree is the ticket to the good life in corporate America. So, with the M.B.A.s and "exciting" concepts such as operations research techniques for forecasting demand, marketing plans for assessing needs or stimulating demand, and organizational development for straightening out the errant firm (or strategic planning for making the most of the competitive environment), we have seen Chrysler almost fold up, Lockheed need a federal bailout, the Pennsylvania Railroad go bankrupt, W.T. Grant go out of business, and countless other firms run into serious trouble.

In the search for a solution, industry has been forced, by competitive circumstances, to turn its attention to the island republic of Japan. Half way around the world, and comprising four main and almost 4,000 smaller islands, Japan is the fifth most densely populated country in the world, with its 118 million people living on approximately 30 percent of its 144,000 square miles. This nation, with a distinct lack of critical natural resources, imports 87 percent of its energy, 81 percent of its wheat, and 92 percent of its food stuff. But the attention of U.S. industry did not turn to Japan because of its imports, but because of its exports. In particular, the U.S. industrial giants were concerned about the numbers of Datsuns and Toyotas on the road, the Sonys and Panasonics in the homes, the Minoltas and Nikons on the shoulders, and the Japanese steel in buildings, elevators, and countless other products. In a generation, Japanese products have progressed from being perceived as cheap and flimsy to being esteemed for their high quality.

At first, the explanation for all of this seemed relatively simple—the Japanese were exploiting their work force: Japanese workers were making less money than their U.S. counterparts. The slogan "Buy American" was heard once again. Driving a Toyota was un-American, and in Detroit it could be dangerous.

Then, as America entered the eighth decade of the twentieth century, two management books were published that touched some sensitive nerves. Both books made the New York Times bestsellers' list, unusual for management books, and particularly unusual in that one of the volumes stayed on the list for several months and was published by a firm that specialized in textbooks. The authors of these popular books were management professors: William Ouchi of the Los Angeles Graduate School of Business at the University of California (author of *Theory Z*) and Richard Tanner Pascale of the Stanford University Graduate School of Business and Anthony Athos of the Harvard University Graduate School of Business Administration (authors of *The Art of Japanese Management*). While each book took a slightly different tack, the theme of each was similar: Japanese industry is winning the race to the consumer's pocketbook, because Japanese industry is better managed. Management, not exploitation or magic, is the key, and in their books the authors demonstrated how that management works in Japan and how it could, and has been, applied in a limited way in the United States.

While the work of Ouchi, Pascale, and Athos has received considerable publicity and notoriety, it must be recognized that articles on Japanese management have appeared for years in the professional literature, but until recently they have been almost ignored. What is perhaps of greater importance is that high-quality research on industrial management in Japan, primarily focusing on the activities of industrial and trading companies, *has* been carried out and reported on for decades.

What relevance does all of this have to hospital administration in the United States? As anyone involved in hospital administration in this country will quickly point out, hospital administration is not the same as industrial management. There are some very significant differences: the nonprofit nature of a significant portion of the hospital industry; the problem of physicians being "off" the organizational chart yet controlling the utilization of an institution's resources; and a rather complicated, some argue archaic, reimbursement system. Some summarize these problems as a lack of a "clear bottom line."

However, some perceived value to the Japanese approach to management must already exist. If it did not, the "QC" (quality circle) sales people would not be in business. Indeed, the phenomenon of American voluntary hospitals going into the subsidiary business of peddling quality circle programs at outrageous rates must suggest need at some level.

Yet, while the Japanese management approach becomes very attractive to those faced with the problems of administering hospitals, a critical question still arises: How is the Japanese approach to industrial management translated into the management of Japanese hospitals? To consider this question we must look at Japan, the Japanese health system, the Japanese hospital scene, and finally, management inside the Japanese hospital. From such an analysis we might be able to develop a model of what might be valuable for utilization in the United States.

It should be clear that this book is primarily written for hospital administrators, board members, medical staffs, and nursing staffs. Other health services administrators, "medical careniks," health care researchers, and Japan scholars will likely find parts of this volume of interest and value—but this book is mainly an attempt to find practical solutions to practical problems by carefully studying the aforementioned questions. It is my hope that readers of this volume will consider the adaptation of *Theory Z,* or any of its components, particularly quality circles, with more care and thought than they would have had they not read this book. For Japanese colleagues this book will serve as one American's impressions and analysis of their approach to hospital management, and perhaps such a review by a foreigner may be beneficial to those interested in change.

My approach to studying the issues of Japanese management, the Japanese health system, and Japanese hospital management used several methods, including a review of the English language literature, field visits, interviews with Japanese physicians, administrators, nurses and hospital staffs, interviews with Japanese health care researchers, interviews with American Japan scholars, and finally, a comparative survey of hospital workers in the United States and Japan. This volume is an analysis and distillation of all those experiences.

As will be obvious, this analysis is biased and limited in a variety of ways, ranging from technical issues involving the survey to my own views of the American health and hospital system and the barriers of socialization, language, and culture. I am not a Japan scholar, nor do I pretend to have the expertise of one. No doubt, some of my observations or analyses about Japan and health care in Japan are inaccurate. For those shortcomings, I apologize. On the other hand, I am one of the growing number of American academics with expertise in some field other than Japan studies who are now attempting to undertake similar discipline-based studies in Japan. I would like to believe that my general openness to new ideas and the earlier experiences of living and working in the Philippines for almost two years, plus my four trips to Japan, various attempts to broaden my intellectual and emotional understanding of Japan, two decades of experience as a hospital administrator, educator, and researcher, and finally, the great help of Japanese colleagues and American East Asian scholars will compensate in some measure for these earlier noted limitations.

Seth B. Goldsmith, Sc.D.

Acknowledgments

Unfortunately, because of confidentiality, there are a number of people to whom I am quite grateful but to whom I cannot acknowledge my debt. There are, however, a number of people and organizations whom I can identify, and I would like to thank them for their contributions to this project.

When I first became interested in this study, several colleagues from the Five College community were most helpful in pointing me toward the relevant literature and providing intellectual support for this endeavor. Professor Jon Lipman of Mount Holyoke College, Professor Richard Minear of the University of Massachusetts, and Professor Emeritus John Maki of the University of Massachusetts were of enormous help. Dr. Joel Broida, who was then with the National Center for Health Services Research, suggested names and literature to follow up on. Dr. Linda Aiken of the Robert Wood Johnson Foundation provided insights from her own visit and suggested relevant literature on nursing. Dr. David Finkelstein and Carl Greene, formerly of the Ford Foundation, provided useful assistance at the beginning stages of this work. A special thanks is particularly accorded to Dr. Finkelstein, whose encouragement and advice made the final trip feasible. My colleagues in the Program in Health Administration, Robert Gage, Jane Zapka, Roger Kropf, and Paula Stamps, provided an important sounding board for my ideas and put up with the problems of an occasionally absent chairman. Bob Gage's insights into Japan were particularly useful. Anne Stoddard's statistical consultations on various aspects of the survey chapter were of great value. Dean William Darity's support and encouragement were crucial and are appreciated.

As anyone who has worked in Japan knows, having the ''right'' sponsors is half the battle. My guardian angels in Japan made the project feasible: without their assistance I would still be standing in line at Narita Airport. My sincerest thanks to Dr. Masakazu Kurata, dean of the School of Medicine at Keio University, and Dr. Teruhiko Saburi, Director General of the National Institute of Hospital Administration. Two individuals on their respective staffs played a crucial role in my work, Masahira Anesaki and Naoki Ikegami, M.D., who deserve a very special thanks for all of their time and effort. Dr. Ikegami's additional contributions as co-author of one chapter and author of an appended bibliography are especially appreciated. At St. Luke's International Hospital, Dr. Tokuro Nobechi provided me with unlimited access, invaluable time, and genuine kindness for which I am grateful. Mr. Kaubayashi and Tekenori Seki deserve special thanks for taking such good care of me. Also, a thanks to Toshiaki Saito for his useful information and good spirits.

Over the course of my travels I met numerous people who also helped me in one way or another. The following is only a very partial list of these people—to those I left out, I apologize—Hirotugu Sawasaki, Dr. Kasuga, Masako Ozeki, Torao Tukuda, Takuo Matsuba, Hisayoshi Miyajima, Kenzo Kiikuni, Tadayuki Maehara, Yoshio Tsumuji, Hiroshi Miyake, Kozo Nishimura, Shogo Nakamura, Eiko Tamura, Kazuhiko Miura, Eugene Aksenoff, Jonathan and Julie Maltzman, Hirotugu Sawasaki, Nobuo Maeda, Barbara Newton, Kiyoshi Matsuura, Tohru Omoi, David Stark, Elyse Rogers, Minoro Kohno, Yukio Konichi, Osamu Doi, Takeo Doi, and the excellent staff of the International House of Japan.

A special thanks is due Dr. Hideoki Ogawa, professor and chairman of the Department of Dermatology at Juntendo University Medical School, who on more than one occasion was generous with his time and expertise. I also wish to thank my brother Lowell A. Goldsmith, M.D., chairman of the Department of Dermatology at the University of Rochester Medical School, who shared with me his own Japanese experiences and contacts.

The International House of Japan became a special place for me to carry on discussions and dialogues about my work with many colleagues, in particular Roger Bowen of Colby College, Dr. and Mrs. Mike Cahn of San Francisco State University, William Foote Whyte of Cornell University, and Ian Kerr of the University of Sussex. Not to be forgotten is William Steslicke, Ph.D. To Bill goes a special thanks for his time and efforts on my behalf. From Bill Steslicke I learned about Japan and collegial relationships—two valued gifts.

To the various anonymous and not-so-anonymous readers and critics of earlier drafts of sections of the manuscript, including some who were previously mentioned, plus Steve Shortell of Northwestern University, John Simmons, author of *Working Together,* Dr. Richard Pierson, Vivian Godbey, Rev. Sam Van Culin and Gary Gambuti—thanks.

Funding for this project came from a patchwork of sources, and to them I wish to express my sincere appreciation. These various groups included the Episcopal Church, World Mission in Church and Society, the University of Massachusetts, Amherst Associates, Chicago, Illinois and Amherst, Massachusetts, and Pan American World Airlines. To those involved with these funding sources, I wish to express my appreciation for their support.

Last, but hardly least, were the contributions of my family. Sandra, busy with her own professional activities, was willing to shoulder the additional burden of a missing spouse. More importantly, she strongly encouraged this project and provided a critical audience for my ideas. Jonas and Benjamin did without their father for three much-too-long periods of time. Our long transcontinental phone calls hardly made up for the absence. Their forebearance while I pursued this study is deeply appreciated.

Seth B. Goldsmith

Part I

Introduction: Problem, Perspective, and Potential

This book is basically an exploration of how hospitals are managed in Japan. In particular, it is about how the Japanese approach to industrial management finds its way into hospital management and what implications the Japanese experience has for the United States. In this section, the background for exploring the problem is developed by first looking at the problems being faced by American hospital management. Obviously, any identification of these problems will be biased in some way, but as one reads through this volume, it is important to understand my perspective on the dilemmas so that the subsequent descriptions and analyses can be put into a proper context.

Next, an overview is presented of Japanese management. This overview, while not an extensive review of the entire literature, does identify the major elements of the Japanese approach to management and will provide the reader with the background necessary to understand the cases and the final discussion about the implications for American hospital management.

The last two chapters in this section focus on Japan. First there is a review of the health system that provides the framework within which hospital management must function, and finally, there is a general description of hospital administration in Japan. What becomes obvious from this section is that there are many striking similarities and differences between our systems of delivering health care and managing those systems. These similarities and differences then set up a challenge: what can we learn from their experiences?

Chapter 1

The American Hospital Dilemma

Hospitals and hospital administrators are caught between the proverbial rock and the hard spot. They are asked to deal in an effective, equitable, and expeditious manner with the problems of health and society, but the means for dealing with these problems are either not provided or taken away. They are asked to control patient or clinical behavior but are not allowed to exercise the authority to implement the controls. In this chapter the stage is set for the remainder of the book by briefly considering some of the uncertainties and problems that hospitals face and then offering a hypothesis for their solution. This background will assist in putting into context the value that the Japanese approach to management has in developing an organization that can effectively operate in the emerging health care environment.

OUT-OF-CONTROL HEALTH CARE COSTS

As the decade of the eighties opened hospitals were faced with severe economic problems. On a national basis the costs of health care approached $300 billion per year, representing almost 10 percent of the gross national product.[1] The largest component of those costs was for hospital care, and this component was growing at an alarming rate. For the federal government, which in the last two decades has become the single largest financer of health care, the problem was critical. Using its leverage over the Medicare and Medicaid programs, the federal government began to design programs that had as their fundamental goal the control of the costs of health care, in particular the costs of providing hospital care. There were many false starts, such as the various proposals to cap capital expenditures, and numerous "experiments" that either did not work or were only partially successful, such as health system agencies and professional standard review organizations. But

3

what is obvious to any observer of the health care scene is that the federal government is not getting out of the business of trying to control health care expenditures. Someday, one approach, perhaps the diagnostic related groupings (DRGs), will be the "answer." Further, the federal government has now enlisted in its army the state governments, which are now also feeling the impact of health care costs, in particular hospital costs that appear to be out of control. For example, Massachusetts has enacted Chapter 372, a hospital cost control measure. In hospitals across the United States beds are being eliminated, hiring freezes have been instituted, and staffs are being fired in order for hospitals to meet their financial targets.

FINDING WAYS TO SAVE MONEY

It is evident that the focus of government energy is being placed on the inputs to the health and hospital system—and these inputs are relatively narrowly defined as money. The theory, if one exists, must be that if one wishes to save money in delivering health services it can be best accomplished by paying the provider less. This would not be a problem if several other elements did not come into play, such as new and costly innovations—or, in the jargon of our day—the intensity of services. A second element is the omnipresent inflation, a third element is the changing disease pattern, a fourth is demography, and a fifth is the ethical issue of equitable access. Thus no matter how you slice the pie delivering health services is going to become more costly. This leads government into experimenting with new ways to limit and save money.

The position of this book is that the focus of government is too much on the input or revenue side of the equation and not enough on the internal organization process part of the problem. Indeed as some evidence for these assertions one can simply look at the fiscal 1984 through 1988 budget proposals of the federal government and see that the major dollar savings will come from increasing the patients' copayment requirements, paying the hospitals on a fixed rate per case basis, paying the doctors on a scheduled basis, increasing patients' premiums for health insurance, and cutting Medicaid matching funds to the states.

THE BURDEN ON THE HOSPITALS

Strangely enough, all of this financial pressure is being placed on hospitals during a period when they are also being asked to redefine their mission—to take a greater responsibility for the total health care in the community and to respond to shifting demographic and disease patterns, by changing from institutions that simply provide patients with care for acute illnesses to ones that provide patients care for the acute episodes of chronic diseases and often the follow-up care for those diseases.

Staffing Problems

Central to the financial problems facing hospitals is the role of the medical staff in decision making, the lack of input others have in the decision making, and the net results of this situation, in particular staffing problems. After looking into the issue of physician involvement in decision making and health care costs, the U.S. General Accounting Office made the following observations in a report issued in 1982:

> The more than 400,000 practicing physicians occupy a unique position in the health care system. In addition to diagnosing illnesses and providing medical care and treatment to patients, physicians also serve as patients' advisors and purchasing agents for health care services that they do not provide themselves. In most cases, physicians determine who goes to the hospital, how long they stay and what diagnostic and treatment services they receive. Physicians exercise similar control over outpatient care, including prescriptions. Consequently, in this decision making role, physicians have wide latitude in determining the type and quantity of care patients receive and the settings in which they receive it. Of necessity, patients rely on physicians for these and other medical decisions.
>
> The physicians' collective decisions significantly affect the national demand and utilization of medical resources. It has been estimated that 70 percent of all expenditures for health care are directly influenced, if not controlled, by the decisions of physicians.[2]

So while medical staffs were busy making expensive decisions, hospitals and their administrators throughout the country were facing serious staffing problems, in particular, the nursing shortage. In responding to these problems new strategies were developed to recruit nursing and other critical staff personnel. Bonuses, child care centers, schedules whereby a nurse could work two extended shifts on weekends and earn a week's pay, and other gimmicks were developed. Newspapers were filled with advertisements touting the virtues of various locations. Some institutions offered bonuses for nurses who recruited other nurses. Hospitals started refresher courses to bring nurses back into nursing. A yearly turnover of 40 percent was not unusual, and the literature was replete with statistical analyses of turnover as well as ways to reduce it. But the one strategy not developed was the one that would give nurses or others in the hospital genuine power in the decision-making process.

The problems of staff productivity also became the subject of popular debate. Seminars were developed to help beleaguered administrators deal with the problem of a poorly motivated work force with high turnover. Alienation of workers from management and institutions continued, and the interest and trend in unionization, particularly professional unionization, did not abate.

As the decade progressed the recession deepened and the unemployment figures in America became staggering. Suddenly any job seemed like a good one, and many hospitals were in the unusual position of being in the driver's seat, with nursing and other staff turnover rates greatly diminished. But the problems of productivity and worker alienation did not abate simply because people did not quit jobs. Indeed, one can foresee two problems on the horizon: First, as the economy improves we will be back to the same old problems of high turnover and its partner of lost investments in the training and development of staff. If the economy does not improve, hospitals will be saddled with disgruntled employees—the selfsame persons who in previous years would have dealt with their frustrations by leaving the organization are now forced to stay because of economics, and they will take out their frustrations in time-honored ways: low productivity, grievances, and absenteeism.

How serious are these staff or human resource management problems? It is suggested here that these problems are quite serious and a fundamental restructuring of relationships is necessary if health care and hospital organizations are going to survive in their present forms. To illustrate this point, it is useful to consider the organization of a nonprofit community hospital. Typically such hospitals have voluntary medical staffs, that is, physicians who are associated with the hospital but who do not derive any of their income directly from the hospital. For decades many of these hospitals have had exclusive contracts with groups of radiologists and pathologists to provide radiology and pathology services. Frequently small groups of anesthesiologists have controlled a part of the operating room. More recently groups of physicians have been enfranchised to run emergency departments.

Despite the appearance of some full-time medical staff the reality has been that most of the medical staff has been off the organization chart—or at least on the side of it. But, it is clear, as noted earlier, that despite their position on a piece of paper the physicians have wielded enormous power. Why? Simply because they have been the ones responsible for generating the revenues that make the organization function. Without the physicians admitting their patients or utilizing the ancillary services for their patients, the organization would be out of business. On the other hand, those people who are on the organization chart, such as nurses and technicians, are relatively powerless, and they know it!

HOSPITAL BOARDS—REAL OR IMAGINARY POWER?

Theoretically, though, the physicians have only limited organizational power, since the legal power is in the hands of the trustees or boards of directors, groups that, Peter Drucker notes, all have one thing in common, ineffectiveness.[3] This board is a nonpaid voluntary group of people, usually elite members of a community who participate as a public good. No doubt they are genuinely concerned about the well-being of the community, but in short order they can easily be co-opted to the point of believing that the well-being of the hospital and the well-being of the community are synonymous, and the best judges of "well-being" are the medical staff.

While board presidents often devote enormous time to their functions, typically board members are called upon only for periodic meetings. Boards usually do not have technical staff readily available, and frequently they are called upon to make decisions with only limited information or a limited amount of time to study information. No wonder they look to those with technical expertise for advice and counsel. In some respects the hospital board member is similar to a member of Congress who must make important policy decisions by relying on the technical expertise of staff, or bureaucrats in operating agencies.

THE PROBLEM WITH ADMINISTRATORS

One of the most important decisions the board makes is the hiring of the organization's top executives. Theoretically these executives are the agents of the boards and should work closely with them. But in reality tension often develops as the executive tries to move an organization in one direction, the medical staff another, and the board becomes interested in understanding what is going on. The net result of this situation is considerable stress and alienation in the board rooms and executive suites of many hospitals. Indeed, hospital executives are retiring early, being fired, and leaving the field in alarming numbers. In a recent publication Witt Associates gave some straight advice to hospital executives: "Because of the increased stress and pressure experienced in today's competitive environment, it seems especially important for long-term CEOs to remain sensitive to their board and medical staff relationships, maintaining a "textbook" perfection in this area."[4] How strange and sad it is that long-term CEOs live in such unstable situations that they must behave with "textbook perfection."

Thus, while presumably the hospital administrator is empowered to carry out the board's policies, the policies themselves have a built-in degree of ambiguity, leaving the administrator in the uncomfortable position of carrying out a policy that he or she did not support, with the less-than-enthusiastic support of the board.

Illustrative of this is the problem of hospitals not reporting physician misconduct. In New York State the health commissioner has put the hospitals on notice that charges will be brought against those that failed to live up to their responsibility of reporting incompetent physicians.[5] Why have hospitals not acted responsibly in the past? Why have hospital administrators, many of them fully cognizant of serious problems, not allowed such matters to be handled outside the institutions? The traditional answers of "not washing dirty laundry in public" or "it would be damaging to the institution" are less than satisfactory. One must wonder about personal executive motivation. To what extent is fear of losing one's job or one's perceived authority at stake? These are difficult but critical questions.

Avoiding Decision Making

All too often managers will take careful steps to avoid controversial decisions—and then proudly proclaim their skills as politicians. Examples abound of administrators who have failed to take the initiative to develop programs that would have enhanced the hospital's viability in the long run but which, over the short term, would have pitted them in a battle with vocal elements of the medical staff. A hospital administrator who is worth his or her salary should be willing to take the tough stands. The hospital administrator is at the crossroads of the organization, where he or she can analyze what is going on in the community, the region, and the hospital and make decisions or at least recommendations for development that the staff surgeon—who, despite a six-figure income and technical expertise—simply does not know about. Yet that surgeon or internist, who is essentially a small businessman, has inordinate power because of the administrator's unwillingness to exert his or her influence and take the risk of "being fired."

It is my contention that health care executives, in particular hospital administrators, have a great deal of unused power and to make use of that power they must get back into the people management business. The most important function a hospital administrator can perform is to influence other people. The source of influence is one's ability to inspire, that is, to lead. One becomes a leader by having a vision of the future, having a vision of where the organization can fit into that future, and understanding how the organization can get from point A to point B.

SOLUTIONS

This book suggests in a variety of ways that the principal way of leading hospitals out of their present morass is *not* in focusing so heavily on the inputs, that is, new and clever schemes of increasing the patient's share of the bill or reducing the dollars the government or insurers pay hospitals. Rather, management should focus greater energy on internal management, specifically the work relationships within hospitals. Not until we can get the 4 million hospital workers to invest themselves in their work, and not until we can reorganize the power structure so that the nurse with 15 years of experience has at least as much say in the future of the hospital as the wet-behind-the-ears physician, will we get off the roller coaster of problems on which we are presently riding.

CONCLUSIONS

When one thinks of the staffing problems in hospitals, it becomes painfully obvious that despite the closing gap between the functions and education of the medical staff and technical staff the power equation has remained the same, and the treatment accorded the different staff groups is disparate. Illustrative of this is a large medical center that has two entrances for staff, one for physicians and one for everyone else. When the medical doctors walk in they encounter a computer screen that asks them to type in their identification number. Up on the screen comes any messages plus an update on the hospital's census, broken down by service. Presumably the computer could also provide information on meetings and perhaps the day's lunch menu. In sharp contrast to this is the employees' entrance, where staff members are greeted with a punch clock, racks of time cards, a TV camera monitoring the entrance, and a bulletin board with out-of-date federal notices. For employees who will spend the next eight hours of their life in that hospital, there is no information about what is going on that day. Is it any wonder that employees are alienated? Finally, despite new technology and changing disease patterns, staffing ratios and the budget slice devoted to manpower have not decreased; indeed, staffing ratios have increased. The explanations for why the power equation has not changed are myriad, ranging from sexist to legal interpretations.

Regardless of the explanations, the conclusions must be the same. This volume focuses on a new path; it is the path of more cooperative work arrangements. This book does not in any way, shape, or form ask for a wholesale importation. Indeed, the cases in this book point up serious weaknesses with the Japanese approach. But what does come through are a set of ideas that, in this author's judgment, would put managers back into management and develop a more balanced organization— one that could be more productive for the community and satisfying for the individual.

NOTES

1. *Health Care Financing Trends,* Health Care Financing Administration (Washington, D.C.: U.S. Government Printing Office), March 1982.
2. *Physician Cost Containment Training Can Reduce Medical Costs,* U.S. General Accounting Office (Washington, D.C.: U.S. Government Printing Office), February 4, 1982.
3. Peter Drucker, *Management* (New York: Harper & Row, 1973), pp. 627–636.
4. Witt Associates, *Perspectives,* no. 6 (Oakbrook, Ill.: Witt Associates, March 1983), p. 1.
5. *New York Times,* April 3, 1983, pp. 1 and 30.

Chapter 2

Management: The Japanese Way

INTRODUCTION

Periodically American managers and students of management look abroad for solutions to their managerial problems. Not too many years ago it was the factories of Sweden and at times the British who were considered to have the answers. Lately, the focus of managerial attention is on Japan. According to a number of commentators, the Japanese have a magic formula that, when applied to ailing American industry and government, will solve the problems of alienation, turnover, and productivity.[1,2,3]

THE MAGIC POTION OF JAPANESE MANAGERIAL SUCCESS

The "magic potion" that has become popularized in America boils down to the following elements: lifetime employment; a company concern for the employees' total well-being; consensus decision making; the development of company-oriented generalist managers rather than professionally oriented specialists, a steady, but by American standards slow, system of promotions with little formal evaluation; and an organizational orientation toward the long run.[4,5,6] Some observers credit the great successes of the Japanese to their managerial approach and, in explaining it, point out that its history dates back to the samurai and Confucius.[7,8] Of course, they do not explain why these approaches, now credited with a tightly organized and productive industrial machine producing first-quality goods, also gave the world, during an earlier period, poor quality and technologically unsophisticated merchandise. It is suggested that using historical antecedents as explanations for the present day successes of Japan is akin to invoking the Puritan ethic in America—full of nostalgia but hardly enlightening.

STEREOTYPING JAPANESE INDUSTRY

In this chapter the concepts that appear to be the bulwark of Japanese management will be examined. However, before examining them we must recognize some important facts about Japanese industry, the literature on Japanese management, and about ourselves. The Tofflers, long-time observers and analysts of Japan, note that Americans tend to view Japan in a stereotypic fashion, seeing a nation of "115,000,000 docile, dedicated and highly motivated workers smoothly managed by a few giant paternalistic corporations whose top leaders work hand in glove with an understanding government."[9] This simplistic characterization of the Japanese, they note, is also a dangerous building block for racism. Indeed, in the wake of the difficult economic times in the United States and the apparently healthy economy in Japan, there have been a number of articles that indicate the development of an anti-Japanese sentiment, in part, making the case that Japan is an exploiter, rather than an excellent manager, of its labor resources.[10,11,12]

JAPAN, INC.: DOES IT EXIST?

The literature that tells the story of the amazing success of "Japan, Inc.," focuses on the largest industries in Japan, often the world-wide trading companies. The examples offered are the Sony Corporation, Toyota, Mitsui, Mitsubishi, or Matstushita. In fact, Japanese industry is primarily made up of smaller business organizations. For example, in 1978 there were 841,000 manufacturing firms employing 12.5 million people. Three-quarters of these firms employed less than 10 people, and slightly under 2 percent of these firms employed more than 100 workers (compared to the United States, where about 11 percent of the manufacturing firms employ more than 100 workers). In Japan, 41.7 percent of the manufacturing work force labor in the large (over 100-employee) firms, but in the United States approximately 75 percent of the work force is employed in firms with more than 100 employees. Another way to demonstrate that Japan is essentially a nation of small businesses is to examine the data on domestic trade. These data indicate that there are 2.8 million commercial businesses in Japan, with 60 percent in the retail trade; 13 percent in the wholesale trade; and 26.5 percent in food services. Almost three-quarters of these businesses (excluding food services) employ less than 5 workers.[13] The image one gets is that of neighborhood industry. Commenting on this situation, a government report concludes: "Japanese domestic trade is characterized by a high percentage of these small-scale businesses, most of which are clustered in shopping streets or shopping centers which are conveniently located close by residential areas."[14]

These points concerning the size of Japanese industry become increasingly important when one realizes that the magic of Japanese management is not evenly diffused throughout the system. For example, quality circles are most likely to be found in the largest corporations and as Woronoff, a well-known commentator on the Japanese scene notes, productivity increases appear to be a function of size, with the largest companies doing considerably better than the smaller ones. Further, he notes that between 1970 and 1978 there has been a decline in productivity in the service sector of the economy.[15]

THE JAPANESE LABOR SCENE

Unionization

In the literature on Japanese management one often sees commentary on the close relationships between unions and management, and while this is often the case, it is also worth remembering that most of the 40 million members of the Japanese work force are not unionized. In 1971 34.8 percent of the work force was unionized (compared with 30.8 percent in 1981). This compares with estimates from the United States, where 24 percent of the work force was unionized (1978); West Germany, with 42 percent unionized (1979); and the United Kingdom, with 57.5 percent unionized (1978).[16,17] An additional perspective on union membership is presented by Cole, who observes that union membership varies by size of the firm: "In Japanese firms of 1000 or more employees some 57 percent of the employees are organized: this compares to a rate of unionization of only 9.3 percent in those firms with 500-900 employees."[18] Cole also points out that union membership is higher in Japan among white collar employees than in the United States.

Enterprise Unions

Perhaps what is most interesting about Japanese unions is their tradition of enterprise unions. Basically the enterprise union is a company-specific union that evolved after the Second World War. The enterprise union, as Cole defines it, has membership from both the blue and white collar work force as well as temporary and regular employees. Membership is automatic upon joining the company, and the union officers are elected by the membership, paid their salary by the union, but always retain their company employee status. This, Cole suggests, results in union officials seeing "their union activities as an opportunity to provide service to the company and a means of enhancing their promotion opportunities."[19] Indeed evidence of this assertion is found in an information bulletin from the Ministry of Foreign Affairs, which points out that in a survey of 313 large corporations, 16.2 percent of the executives were former union leaders.[20]

But it should be noted that the Japanese labor relations situation is not without its ups and downs. A review of Table 2-1 on page 23, which provides comparative statistics for the United States and Japan, will indicate that there have been good and bad years for labor disputes, work stoppages, and lost days of production.

So, in thinking about Japan, we must also factor into our equation the information that 69 percent of the work force is not unionized and, in some senses, not protected by collective bargaining agreements and that the union has a company- as opposed to industry-wide focus—a focus that, as will be demonstrated in one subsequent case, causes the union to identify strongly with the success of the organization.

A Homogeneous Work Force

A second crucial point to consider is that the Japanese are, for the most part, dealing with an ethnically homogeneous work force. The Japanese work force is almost entirely Japanese, virtually every member having been born in Japan, having had a similar, standardized primary school education, and having been socialized to the values, attitudes, and beliefs of the Japanese society and family. Consider the implications of the following data: Between 1972 and 1980 the number of divorces has increased from 108,000 to 142,000, giving Japan a divorce rate of under one percent—one of the lowest in the developed world.[21] By comparison, in 1979 there were 1,181,000 divorces in the United States.[22] Thus for the Japanese youngster, who eventually becomes the Japanese worker, the years of childhood will be with an intact family and an employed father and more likely than not, the full-time attention of a mother. Religiously, the Japanese share their Buddhist or Shinto religions as well as their range of secular holidays. All of this is in sharp contrast to the United States, where the production work forces, and to some extent the managerial work forces, particularly in hospitals, come from all social classes, ethnic backgrounds, and frequently, foreign countries. The mosaic society of America is reflected in its work force and the managerial problems that are encountered.

Recently some Japanese companies have gained first-hand experience with the problems of a heterogeneous work force because they have opened production facilities in the United States. The Japanese have encountered a range of difficulties as the two cultures have come into contact with one another. In some instances the Japanese branch manager has difficulty making the home office understand the American way of relating to employees, and in other instances the Japanese manager must make significant stylistic adjustments in order to manage in this country. It is suggested that the task of managing people with a shared socialization and value system is easier (and certainly less challenging) than the task of managing a work group comprising people from different social classes.

A third point is that there is *not* something called Japan, Inc. The idea that government and industry are happily marching down the street together, both holding hands with labor, is a simplistic overstatement. As Drucker points out, the Japanese government has not been able to get the computer manufacturers to pool their resources, and there is considerable competition in Japan for both the domestic and foreign markets.[23] Put simply, whether it is cars or computers, Japan is not one big happy family.

THE ELEMENTS OF JAPANESE MANAGERIAL SUCCESS

Now we shall turn our attention to the five elements that are allegedly the secret of Japanese managerial success.

Lifetime Employment

The first of these elements is lifetime or permanent employment. To begin, it is clear from the literature and interviews that the Japanese company hires most of its staff with the intention that those hired will be permanent employees. However, this concept, as most westerners understand it, is grossly oversimplified. For example, lifetime employment defines lifetime in a rather narrow sense, normally from the time of first hiring (somewhere between ages 18 and 24) to the retirement age of 55. In actual practice we are usually talking about a 30-year contract—for the most productive thirty years of one's life.[24] After 55, in most cases, workers receive a lump sum payment, usually equal to one month's pay for each year of service, and are off on their own. With life expectancies in excess of 70 for males and 75 for females, there is still plenty of life that the company isn't concerning itself with in its lifetime employment approach. But to one important commentator, Tadashi Hanami, professor of law and dean of the School of Law at Sophia University, lifetime employment is a powerful force and one that ensures "strong loyalty to and identification with their enterprise. Since they stay in the same enterprise for their entire working lives, their fate and well being depend almost entirely on the prosperity of the enterprise."[25]

A second point of significance is that the Japanese work force is divided into two groups: the permanent employees and the temporary employees. The latter group, representing an estimated 20 percent of the work force, does not have lifetime employment status. Females, as a category of worker, are also usually excluded from the permanent employee category. All of this does not preclude a company from discharging temporary employees and temporarily laying off permanent employees or shifting them to other parts of the firm. There are numerous stories in literature describing how companies have sent their production workers into the field to sell the companies' products to stimulate demand or how top executives' salaries were cut to save the jobs of workers.

Another side to the lifetime employment question is the perspective of the potential employee. In a study of graduating male college seniors, the Nippon Recruit Center found that 69.4 percent of those surveyed expected to work for the same company until retirement; 8.6 percent thought they would change employers; and 21.7 percent thought that eventually they would go into business for themselves.[26] In short, lifetime employment in Japan is a situation where both employers and employees expect a long-term commitment to the organization and can act on that commitment in making personal and personnel investments.

Holistic Concern for the Employee

The second element of Japanese managerial success is a concern for the total welfare of the employee. This concern is evidenced by the provision of company housing and a wide range of social programs for employees including sports and cultural clubs, health benefits, retirement programs, vacation resorts, and almost anything else that can be conjured up. In discussing this attitude of wholism, Chie Nakane wrote in her seminal work that new employees "were trained by the company not only technically but also morally. In Japan it has always been believed that individual moral and mental attitudes have an important bearing on productive power."[27] For those of us who have spent any number of years in the armed forces, particularly on remote foreign duty stations, the wholistic approach of the Japanese company is strikingly familiar. The folklore of Japanese management is full of stories about corporations inducting new employees into the firm with the parents of the new employees essentially turning their children over to the company as *locum parentis*. While I did not observe any such dramatic activity in hospitals, this text will show the strength of the commitment made to the new employee, as evidenced by programs such as the intensive orientation periods. Is this typical of America? Again, the military analogy is apt: think of the drama of the commissioning, promotion, or awards ceremonies or the "birthday parties" held each year for the services or even the units in the services. For example, there is the tradition of the annual MSC birthday party in the Navy, where hundreds of officers share an evening of celebration ostensibly to celebrate the birthday of the founding of the medical service corps.

Worker Orientation Periods

One important development of this wholistic concern is the general practice among Japanese companies of hiring employees once a year and providing an orientation, often in the neighborhood of 10 days, to the entire group. This practice accomplishes three purposes: it develops "team" spirit, it builds a support network among all new employees who begin their working careers at the same time, and it allows the company to invest more heavily in orientation because it occurs only once a year.

Orientation serves many purposes. It is a mechanism for fostering loyalty as well as a means for establishing the rankings of the various staff within the organization. By the end of the orientation period each new employee clearly knows the pecking order—a very important factor if one is to function both effectively and politely in the Japanese organization. The net result of this total involvement of the company in the life of the employee is a significantly different relationship between Japanese workers and supervisors than between their American counterparts.

Attitudes of American versus Japanese Factory Workers

Perhaps the clearest illustration of this difference in attitudes was demonstrated in the research project of Takezawa and Whitehill, in which they compared the attitudes and opinions of Japanese and American factory workers.[28] In one question workers were asked if they thought their supervisor should be involved in their marriage plans. Of the U.S. workers, 74 percent thought the supervisor should not be involved in the plans; in contrast, among the Japanese workers, only 5 percent thought the supervisor shouldn't be involved.[29] Another question in the survey asked whether an employee who is feeling well should offer his or her seat to an immediate supervisor who boards the same bus. Thirty-two percent of the Japanese workers, but only 5 percent of the American workers, replied affirmatively.[30] In a question about the company providing subsidized housing, 47 percent of the Japanese workers, but only 7 percent of the American workers, agreed that this was something the company should do.[31] A final question touched on the issue of extracurricular activities: "With reference to baseball games, picnics or overnight excursions for workers, it is best for the company to plan such activities for workers, but leave participation strictly voluntary." Sixty-one percent of the American workers, but only 14 percent of the Japanese workers, agreed with this statement.[32] This research, as well as other studies, reveals fundamental differences in how the worker perceives the role of the company, and the behavior of the company reveals fundamental differences in its concept of how it relates to, and invests in, its employees.[33,34]

Consensus Decision Making

A third element in the formula of Japanese managerial success is collective or consensus type decision making, or, in Japanese, *ringi-seido*. This, as Gibney points out, is the "bottom-up initiative as opposed to the top-down direction."[35] In reviewing this approach Gibney describes the slow process of a document passing through various organizational layers, being reviewed and commented upon and eventually passing, with modification and approval, to the next organizational level so that by the time it reaches the president, "all that is needed is his seal." The net result of this process is a series of commitments at lower levels through involvement in the decision-making process; clarification of the human and material resources necessary to effect the process; and assurances that the pieces are in place before the president signs off. The Japanese manager is depicted as a person more concerned with discussing and organizing the details of a decision than the American manager, whose focus appears to be on making the decision, leaving details of its implementation to others. It is as if American managers are most interested in expediency, while the Japanese are more concerned with the effectiveness of implementation.

This approach was well illustrated to me over a pizza in a restaurant in Tokyo. Toward the end of one of my trips I was discussing hospital administration education with a professor from a Japanese university. After reviewing several curriculums, I had what I thought to be a series of reasonable suggestions for change. After offering my ideas, with appropriate politeness and caveats, the discussion moved away from the merit of my ideas to the fundamental issues of implementation. I wished to talk about the value of my conceptualizations; my luncheon partner wanted to talk about the details of implementation. As the discussion evolved, my suggestions were shown to have a limited value because of the realistic details of implementation.

Another military analogy: As a young naval officer I found that even my most brilliant ideas had to be approved by the lieutenant who supervised me, the commander who supervised him, and the captain who supervised all of us. In turn the corpsmen who worked for me required my "chop" on most things before they could move them up the line—despite my being a wet-behind-the-ears ensign. The system, not the people in it, who were essentially interchangeable, dictated the decision process.

The Generalist Approach

The next element in the formula is the generalist as opposed to the specialist approach. The idea here is that Japanese managers spend their careers rotating through the various components of the organization, developing their expertise in the organization itself but not necessarily in a particular part of the organization. Thus someone might work three years in personnel, then be shifted into domestic marketing, and then into finance, etc. The advantages of such a system are clear— management personnel acquire a broad view of the organization, and when decisions are being considered they have the experience to see what is happening from a number of vantage points. Similarly, it means that all staff are tuned into the total system of the corporation. Thus, as is often pointed out, when you call a Japanese business firm and get the wrong department, the person at the other end of the line often knows the answer to your question because that person worked in the other department at some time in his or her career. All of this is somewhat reminiscent of the family unit where people have a good idea of what is happening in one another's lives and sometimes schedules. From a management perspective this approach has some inherent value; however, there are limitations, some of which are illustrated in the Public Corporation case, in Chapter 5.

Amae: Holding It All Together

The glue holding all of this together is the concept of *amae* popularized by the Japanese psychiatrist Takeo Doi in his often quoted book, *The Anatomy of Dependence.*[36] *Amae* is defined by Doi as "an emotion which partakes of the nature of a drive and with something instinctive at its base."[37] He has further defined it as the psychological craving a newborn has for its mother and "the desire to deny the fact of separation that is an inevitable part of human existence, and to obliterate the pain that this separation involves."[38] One observer defined *amae* as "indulgent love" and suggested that it was the central concept in Japanese relationships.[39] According to Gibney, *amae* means literally, "to presume on the affections of someone close to you."[40] Further, he notes that "the *amae* syndrome is pervasive in Japan. It is a mark of this collective society that most of its members expect in some way to be taken care of. The minority who do not expect this have a stern and relatively unprotected role in Japanese life, although to put it mildly, an essential one."[41]

In the organizational setting, the concept of *amae* takes on great significance in that the worker is a dependent of the supervisor. In practice it means that if an employee fails to get promoted, the supervisor views himself as a failure. In America we would simply say, "that's too bad, but it's not my problem," rather than the Japanese style of saying the supervisor "owns the problem." The mutual interdependency that one sees in Japan is sorely lacking in America.

DISADVANTAGES OF THE JAPANESE SYSTEM

Little is said about the disadvantages of the Japanese managerial system. First, however, it precludes anyone from developing depth in any given area. Thus as will be seen in the Public Corporation case, the rotation of managers involves the staff in a process of continually learning a new routine, and just at the point of developing some expertise, moving on to another post. Second, from an American perspective it increases the strain on the employee—the constant job shifting often involves relocation. In the United States we are in the midst of a revolution among management staff concerning relocation. Third, from the managers' perspective it makes them captive to the corporation. After 10 or 15 years with a given corporation all that managers have learned is their company's approach to dealing with a range of issues and problems; they have not developed depth in a specialty that might be valued at another company. Thus the system has the somewhat insidious effect of keeping the employee beholden to the corporation. Contrast this with the American system, where, with the exception of some executive training programs, the young manager goes straight into marketing, personnel, or another specialty and begins to develop expertise in that area. That expertise is readily transferable and marketable to other firms.

PROFESSIONAL VERSUS GROUP IDENTITY

Americans appear more concerned with professional identity, which is, to some extent, an extension of individuality. The Japanese, and granted this is a broad generalization, appear more interested, workwise, in group identity. Thus, the often-cited experience of asking a Japanese what he or she does and hearing a reply such as "I work at Mitsui" is a reflection of this group identity. An American's response is invariably "I am a . . . ," reflecting the striving for a personal or perhaps group identity within a profession but not an organization.

RISING THROUGH THE JAPANESE CORPORATION

The final element to be discussed in this chapter is the issue of slow promotions and evaluation. This element has often been described as the escalator approach. Basically, Japanese managers get on an escalator when they join the firm, and slowly move up the line. At some time (at about age 45) they will be reviewed by the top management, and a decision will be made whether to track them into top management or into the level below. If selected for top management the mandatory retirement age of 55 is waived. If not selected for top management their career with the company will come to an end within the next decade. The literature tells us that the decision is based on a series of informal evaluations made by superiors over a span of years.

All of this again reminds one of an example involving the American military, the promotion of military officers. If you do an outstanding job you are promoted from ensign to lieutenant (junior grade) in a year and a half. If you do a barely adequate job you are promoted in 18 months. The move to the next rank also involves a specific time in rank. Thereafter, time is still a factor but merit becomes increasingly important. The difference between the military—with its structured promotions, job rotation, permanent employment, and regulated retirement ages—and the Japanese organization is the feedback provided by the evaluation schemes. The American military and most American organizations put much emphasis on the need for regular evaluation and feedback to staff about their evaluations. Conversely, Japanese managers may spend most of their career without any direct feedback concerning performance. They will have to pick up—and interpret correctly—subtle clues to know how they are doing. Sometimes, as Drucker points out, a mentor is assigned and the mentor will provide advice and guidance.[42] But without a mentor, managers, essentially bound to their company, may not know where they stand. Some observers say this is why managers spend so much time at the workplace or socializing with colleagues, often skipping vacations or taking them with the "boys"—all in an effort to develop and maintain relationships that are important to a cordial work environment and a secure future.

IMPLICATIONS OF THE JAPANESE SYSTEM

Training and Educating Managers

The implications of all of this are important. For example, each company must essentially be responsible for the training and education of its own managers. For example, Sasaki notes that management training at Toyota consists "of on the job training, off the job programmed education and human relations activities."[43] Sasaki goes on to label this approach as "confined management development," a situation where the manager becomes so organizational specific that he or she is of limited value to the greater marketplace.[44] In Japan we do not see the graduate-level degree in management as the entry ticket into the corporation. Rather it is the college degree—from the right college—which is more important than the major, since the corporation will provide the essential training. Second, as noted earlier, personal relationships are crucial both with colleagues and superiors. Relationships with colleagues are significant because of the family-like atmosphere, and the relationships with superiors are critical if one wishes to advance one's ideas or have a chance for a slot at the top.

Corporate Stability

A third implication is that the corporation is essentially stable. Turnover is low; predictability is high. One knows the chain of command—surprises are few. What this means is that long-range planning can go on in an atmosphere of some certainty and commitment, in sharp contrast to many American organizations. An example of this is a state university where a new chancellor embarked on an 18-month effort to develop a long-range plan. Tens of thousands of dollars and countless hours were invested in his plan, which resulted in a several-hundred-page document. Shortly after its release he announced his resignation. The acting chancellor then essentially scrapped the plan in favor of his own version, which was dramatically shorter. Several months later a new chancellor was appointed, who decided to take another look himself.

The Japanese organization allows people to invest of themselves with some assurance of stability. By the same token the Japanese organization invests in its people, because they know that they are dealing with a stable resource and that the payoff will result in long-term gains. Compare this with the American manager who often seems permanently available for a new job or the American corporation permanently available to hire a new manager, hire from outside, and ready to shift directions.

APPLICATION TO HOSPITALS

Of course, as most hospital administrators are quick to note, hospitals are different from industrial corporations, but how different are they? In the next six chapters that question will be explored, first by considering the context of hospitals in the Japanese health care delivery system and then by looking at hospital management in Japan. Next, three hospital case studies will be presented, and then the results of a cross-cultural study that looked at hospital workers in three Japanese hospitals and three American hospitals will be reviewed.

Table 2-1 Work Stoppages and Their Implications in Japan and the United States

	Japan			United States		
Year	Disputes	Employees Involved (per 1,000 persons)	Workdays Lost (per 1,000 persons)	Disputes	Employees Involved (per 1,000 persons)	Workdays Lost (per 1,000 persons)
1960	1,063	918	4,912	3,333	1,320	19,100
1965	1,542	1,682	5,669	3,963	1,550	23,300
1970	2,260	1,720	3,915	5,716	3,305	66,414
1974	5,211	3,621	9,663	6,074	2,778	47,991
1976	2,720	1,356	3,254	5,648	2,420	37,859
1977	1,712	692	1,518	5,506	2,040	35,822
1978	1,517	660	1,358	4,230	1,623	36,922

Sources: Adapted from *Labour Administration in Japan* (Tokyo: Ministry of Labour, 1980), p. 59; and The U.S. Department of Commerce, *Statistical Abstract of the United States 1982–1983*, Table 684, "Work Stoppages: 1947–1981" (Washington, D.C.): December 1982, p. 410.

NOTES

1. E.F. Vogel, *Japan As Number 1* (New York: Harper Colophon, 1980).
2. P.F. Drucker, "What We Can Learn from Japanese Management," *Harvard Business Review* 59, no. 3 (March–April, 1971): 110–122.
3. P. Patton, "Bringing the Japanese Work Ethic to the U.S.A.," *Pan Am Clipper*, May, 1982, p. 43.
4. W. Ouchi, *Theory Z* (Reading, Mass.: Addison-Wesley, 1981).
5. R.T. Pascale and A.G. Athos, *The Art of Japanese Management* (New York: Simon and Schuster, 1981).
6. R. Hayes, "Why Japanese Factories Work," *Harvard Business Review* 59, no. 4 (July–August, 1981): 57–66.
7. M. Musahi, *The Book of Five Rings—The Real Art of Japanese Management*, trans. Nihon Services Corporation (New York: Bantam Books, 1982).
8. R. Yates, "Japan's Business Excellence Goes to the Roots of Its Culture," *Chicago Tribune*, April 15, 1982.
9. A. Toffler and H. Toffler, "Sifting Facts from Fiction about Number 1," *Japan Times Weekly*, March 7, 1981.
10. "In Ohio, the Enemy is Japan," *New York Times*, April 25, 1982.
11. "Japan as Sneaky Little Yellow People," *Japan Times*, May 19, 1982.
12. S. Kamata, *Japan in the Passing Lane* (New York: Pantheon, 1982).
13. *81 Japan*, Japanese Prime Minister's Office, Statistics Bureau, Tokyo, 1981.
14. Ibid., p. 31.
15. J. Woronoff, *Japan's Wasted Workers* (Tokyo: Lotus Press, 1981), pp. 14–17.
16. "Figuring Out Japan," *Japan Times*, May 5, 1982.
17. "Japanese Labor Unions and 'Shunto'," *Focus Japan*, JSA, JSB, March, 1982.
18. R. Cole, "Enterprise Unions," in *Business and Society in Japan*, ed. B.M. Richarson and Taizo Ueda (N.Y.: Praeger, 1981), pp. 36–37.
19. Ibid., p. 41.
20. "Unions Are Pools for Future Executives," Japanese Ministry of Foreign Affairs, Public Information and Cultural Affairs Bureau, Information Bulletin, Vol 29, no. 1, January 15, 1982.
21. "Divorce in Japan," *Japan Times*, December 14, 1981.
22. U.S. Department of Commerce, Statistical Abstract of the United States, 102nd Edition (Table 124, Marriages and Divorces, 1950-1979), 1981, p. 80.
23. P. Drucker, "Behind Japan's Success," *Harvard Business Review* 59, no. 1 (Jan.–Feb. 1981), pp. 83–90.
24. R. Clark, *The Japanese Company* (New Haven: Yale University Press, 1979), p. 174.
25. T. Hanami, *Labor Relations in Japan* (Tokyo: Kodansha, 1979), p. 28.
26. "Japan's Job Hunting Season," *Focus Japan*, October, 1981, pp. JSA, JSB.
27. Chie Nakane, *Japanese Society* (New York: Penguin, 1970), p. 17.
28. S. Takezawa and A. Whitehill, *Work Ways: Japan and America* (Tokyo: Japan Institute of Labor, 1981).
29. Ibid., pp. 117–121.
30. Ibid., pp. 122–125.

31. Ibid., pp. 157–163.
32. Ibid., pp. 165–171.
33. R. Dore, *British Factory-Japanese Factory* (Berkeley: University of California Press, 1973).
34. R. Cole, *Work, Mobility and Participation* (Berkeley: University of California Press, 1979).
35. F. Gibney, *Japan—The Fragile Superpower* (Tokyo: Tuttle, 1979), p. 215.
36. Takeo Doi, *The Anatomy of Dependence* (Tokyo: Kodansha, 1973).
37. Ibid., p. 166.
38. Ibid., p. 167.
39. B. DeMente, *The Japanese Way of Doing Business* (Englewood Cliffs, N.J.: Prentice-Hall, 1981), pp. 13–17.
40. F. Gibney, *Japan—The Fragile Superpower* (Tokyo: Tuttle, 1979), p. 119.
41. Ibid., p. 120.
42. P. Drucker, "What We Can Learn from the Japanese," *Harvard Business Review* 49, no. 2 (March–April, 1971), pp. 120–121.
43. N. Sasaki, *Management and Industrial Structure in Japan* (Oxford: Pergamon Press, 1981), pp. 40–41.
44. Ibid., p. 47.

Chapter 3

The Japanese Health Service: An Overview*

Naoki Ikegami and Seth B. Goldsmith

Japan has experienced a dramatic improvement in health status indices during the past quarter of a century. The life expectancy at birth has risen from 63.6 years for males and 67.7 years for females in 1955 to 73.3 and 78.8 years, respectively, in 1980. The infant mortality rate has decreased from 39.8 to 7.5 deaths per 1,000 live births.[1] Although the proportion of the gross national product devoted to health care has risen from 3.27 percent to 5 percent, the figure still remains low when compared with most western nations.[2] The improvement in health status indices deserves study and may have relevancy for the health care analyst.

HISTORICAL BACKGROUND

Japan is geographically isolated from the rest of the Eurasian continent and thus was free to develop its own unique culture. This tendency was intensified by a self-imposed policy of isolation that effectively terminated western influence from 1638 to 1854. Two important features of the health care system during this period should be noted. One was the large number of medical practitioners. A census done shortly after this period, in 1871, showed that 86.2 per 100,000 population gave medical practice as their profession, which was remarkably high for a preindustrial society. The majority followed the Chinese school, in which the dispensing of medicine was the most important service. This tradition continues, and dispensing is done in almost all hospitals and clinics. Although a large number of practitioners existed, there was no form of professional organization. This may be interpreted as due to the fact that vertical relationship is more important than

*Reprinted from the *Journal of Ambulatory Care Management,* November, 1982, with permission of Aspen Systems Corporation.

mutual horizontal organizations in all aspects of Japanese society.[3] The other interesting feature was that no institution existed that was similar to the hospital nor any kind of public welfare system offering residential care. These traditions were to have lasting influence in the modeling of health care.[4]

Westernization Influences Health Care

When, in 1868, the Japanese government embarked on a policy of rapid westernization to maintain its national integrity, health care was included as one of the fields to be modernized. The government established medical schools and built accompanying hospitals. From 1883, the granting of licenses was restricted to those who had studied western medicine. The physicians eagerly studied the latest German medicine; conducted research; and, for their convenience, brought their patients to their practice sites. Thus, hospitals in Japan started out not as houses for patients, but as houses for physicians and can be regarded as an outgrowth of living quarters for the outpatients. It was the general custom, until after World War II, for the family of the patient to provide the patient's bedding and food. Nurses were trained by the physicians to provide clinical assistance to the patient, but their inpatient care role was not emphasized. The hospital started from the outpatient department, and inpatient care did not then occupy the dominant position as in western countries.

As medicine developed and clinical specialties progressed, physicians would elect a specialty and perform research within their field. When they opened their own clinics, they had already specialized to some degree; thus, the division into general practitioner and specialist did not occur in Japan. Official board examination similar to that in the United States has never developed, and it is left to the physician to proclaim a specialty when opening a practice. When a position in a hospital becomes vacant, the usual custom is to go to the university with which the hospital is associated and ask the head professor of the vacated specialty to suggest a physician to fill that position. This process still occurs, even in small private hospitals. Thus, the vertical relationship between the teaching hospital and its graduates remains stronger than that of the bond within professional societies. It follows that good positions can usually only be secured by graduates of prestigious universities, as nearly all professors are graduates of the universities in which they teach.

Post–World War II Expansion

After World War II, the occupying forces tried to remodel the hospital according to the western style. They were successful to some degree; however, the medical care law still requires a physician to carry both the final administrative and clinical responsibility and act as both hospital administrator and medical director. During the postwar period of rapid expansion, medical institutions also developed greatly. Some physicians expanded their clinics into hospitals and continuously enlarged their wards. Several new medical schools have grown to that position from their beginnings as clinics within a single generation. Nearly 70 percent of the hospitals are privately owned by physicians. It is imperative for the physician owner of the hospital or clinic to ensure that it stays within the family. It is for this reason that some of the private medical schools can afford to charge high entrance fees, exceeding 20 million yen ($60,000). Medical education in Japan is for the very talented or the very rich.

This historical background has made the difference between the clinic and the hospital less apparent than in western countries. All physicians work full time, either at hospitals or in clinics. Physicians who go into practice to open clinics can very seldom use hospital facilities. All inpatients come through the outpatient department, with the exception of emergency and special cases. As there is little incentive for a practitioner working in a clinic to hospitalize a patient (apart from professional need), referral cases are usually infrequent and, in many cases, the patients visit the hospital on their own initiative. Thus, the health care system could be regarded as giving ambulatory care the dominant position. Further, as the system is presently structured, the hospital must maintain a large ambulatory care service to ensure a flow of inpatients.

HEALTH INSURANCE SYSTEM

Health insurance in Japan had its beginning in 1922, for selected industrial workers. It has gradually expanded so that, by 1961, all Japanese were covered by some kind of compulsory health insurance. At present, for those employed and those over 70 the coverage is 100 percent; for the family of the employed and the self-employed the coverage is 70 percent. However, in the latter groups any self-payment greater than 39,000 yen ($117) is refunded. Although the various insurance schemes have maintained their independent form of funding, third party payment is uniformly based on the *point-fee system*.

The Point-Fee System

The basic concept of this payment scheme is that the fee for each individual service (point) is rigidly and minutely regulated. Thus, for example, the price for an appendectomy is 37,000 yen ($111) regardless of the difficulty of the operation, whether it was performed by an experienced or inexperienced surgeon, or whether it was done in a teaching or a private hospital.[5] The reimbursement is therefore irrespective of the actual cost to the hospital. The point-fee system basically favors reimbursement for material, and service that is difficult to measure is apt to be neglected (e.g., technical expertise).

As Table 3-1 shows, the consultation fee (physicians' service charge) per patient represents .1 percent of total inpatient and 23.3 percent of total outpatient expenditures.[6,7] On the other hand, medication, including injections, still comprises 28.8 percent of the inpatient's and 51.5 percent of the outpatient's bill. The operation figure includes the service fee of the physician.

Although a recent revision has made medical expertise more remunerative, the basic pattern remains the same. There are still professional activities (e.g., group therapy) that are not reimbursed under the system. Such services are usually performed without charge. In spite of these defects, health care without insurance is extremely rare since almost the entire population is covered in whole or in part by some type of health insurance. For example, in Tokyo there is only one clinic exclusively devoted to psychotherapeutic care for private patients.

Table 3-1 Average Composition of the Monthly Insurance Returns per Patient

Treatment	Inpatient 1965	Inpatient 1980	Outpatient 1965	Outpatient 1980
Consultation	.2%	.1%	12.5%	23.3%
Medication	10.4	6.6	51.6	43.9
Injection	20.2	22.2	21.3	7.6
Physical therapy	—	1.0	—	0.7
X-ray diagnosis	2.8	2.3	3.8	4.9
Laboratory examination	4.2	9.1	2.8	12.2
Operation	5.0	5.2	0.5	3.3
Hospitalization	54.1	50.0	—	—
Other	2.9	3.5	7.5	3.6
Total*	100.0	100.0	100.0	100.0

*Rounded to the nearest 10th percentile.

Source: Adapted from the Ministry of Health and Welfare, 1965, 1980.

The fee for an electrocardiogram with 12 leads (including its interpretation) is 1,500 yen ($4.50). If it is only performed using 6 leads, the fee is 900 yen ($2.70). In the case of the electrocardiogram's use in the intensive care unit, 900 yen ($2.70) is charged for every 30 minutes of monitoring; however, from over 8 hours to under 24 hours, there is a flat fee of 15,000 yen ($45). The fee for a hepatic function laboratory examination is 600 yen ($1.80) per test; however, for a combination of examinations, the price decreases as the number of tests increases. The fee for a physician's house call is 2,000 yen ($6); for every visit that is over 2 kilometers (1.2 miles) from the clinic there is an additional charge of 1,000 yen ($3). However, if the physician makes over two calls, the distance is only measured from the house of the former visit. Fees are also predetermined for visits in the evening, during the night, bad weather, to isolated islands, or any combination of these contingencies. A new fee was gradually added to the former fee for individual circumstances that could not be defined exactly.

At the end of each month, the hospitals and clinics submit a bill to the Social Insurance Medical Care Fee Payment Fund. The money from each insurance scheme is pooled, and each bill is checked by a medical jury before payment is made. Part of the fee may be deleted if the medical jury decides that it is too high according to the level of care of the community. The decision is based on the sex, age, and diagnosis of the patient and the medical institution where each bill is from.

Increasing Revenue

It can easily be inferred that there are only two ways for hospitals and clinics to increase their revenue, as it is impossible to pass on the actual cost of the service to the third party. One way is to increase the number of patients and the number of services per patient. The other is to concentrate on the services where the reimbursement is higher than the cost (e.g., medication). It should be remembered that the increase in revenue is of paramount importance to the hospital, since personnel expenses are expected to rise each year in accordance with the general level of wage increases. As the health insurance reimbursement scheme has been one of the most resistant to inflation, the latter is equally important to the hospital administrator. Revision of the fee scale can only be made by the Minister of Health and Welfare acting on the recommendation of the Central Social Insurance Medical Council, which consists of eight representatives of insurers, eight of providers (physicians, dentists, and pharmacists), and four of the public interest. The organization of the committee makes revisions difficult in practice. It has been calculated that while the gross national product has increased 21 times from 1952 to 1975, the fee scale has increased only 2.7 times.[8] The increase in the total health care cost has resulted largely from the increase in the number of patients and the change in the structure of services due to the advancement of medical technology. According to a one-day survey of all medical facilities, the absolute number of inpatients and outpatients has more than doubled from 1955 to 1979.[9,10]

High Patient Volume

Table 3-2 shows the number of patients per physicians and nurses in the various types of medical institutions.[11] It can be seen that they all carry a high volume. Besides the necessity of increasing patient volume, several other reasons contribute to this phenomenon. In the case of inpatients, hospitals in Japan also have the function of intermediate care facilities, so that the intensity of care is not uniformly high. Lengthy consultations are not expected by the patients. Few clinics, with the exception of dental clinics, and a few hospitals have an appointment system.

One result of this health care system is that patients visit their physicians more frequently than in the United States. According to the National Health Survey, 55.7 percent of the population visited a hospital or were hospitalized during the past year.[12] This proportion increased to 79.6 percent for those over age 70. According to a 1980 survey, 9.7 percent of the total population, and 40.2 percent of those over age 70, visited the hospital or were hospitalized for over 31 days. It should be noted that the data from the National Health Survey does not differentiate between inpatients and outpatients. According to the patient survey, 1.0 percent of the general population was hospitalized—and 6.1 percent visited hospitals and clinics—on the surveyed day. This proportion rises to 4.4 percent and 15.3 percent, respectively, for those over age 70.[13] These figures all point to a

---

Table 3-2 Number of Patients per Staff According to Type of Institution

	Hospitals			Clinics	
	Psychiatric	Tuberculosis	General	General	Dental
Physicians/dentists					
Inpatients	42.2	18.2	7.8	—	—
Outpatients	3.8	5.2	12.7	44.7	27.0
Nurses					
Inpatients	6.7	5.9	2.7	—	—
Outpatients	.6	1.7	4.3	49.8	—

Source: Adapted from the Ministry of Health and Welfare, 1979.

high utilization of medical facilities, especially by the elderly. The competition for patients by the medical institutions together with the absolute freedom to visit any physician or institution that the patient desires under the universal health insurance coverage have contributed in part to a practice of early diagnosis and early treatment. On the other hand, the relatively low reimbursement for medical services requiring expertise and expensive technical equipment has discouraged the expanding of facilities into new fields. Since reimbursement frequently does not cover the actual cost of the service, the service is usually provided due to a combination of medical need, professional pride, and the necessity of attracting patients. On the rare occasion, such as in the case of renal dialysis, when there is urgent need to spread a new form of service, reimbursement is initially set very high.

Wide Variation in Fees

To make an extreme contrast, treatment for a common cold at a clinic (including medication for three days, three consultations, and a urine test) would cost 3,520 yen ($10.56). On the other hand, the operation for a ventricular septal defect would be only 250,000 yen ($750) including all material. In addition, as the reimbursement of medication is usually about 20 percent more than the actual price, and since dispensing is almost always done by the clinics and hospitals, the former becomes increasingly attractive. This is reflected in the income that the physicians earn. Generally, the practitioner in the clinic makes more than the practitioner employed by the hospital. Furthermore, the method of taxation makes the practitioner additionally comfortable. Under the previous tax system, practitioners could have a flat 72 percent undetermined deduction of their income. Since 1979, there has been a gradual reduction in the deduction, set according to income level.

PROBLEMS FACING THE FUTURE

The health care system in Japan has its share of problems. The calculation of the total medical care cost differs in each country, and in Japan, it underestimates the costs by not including capital outlay for the construction of public hospitals, extra charge rooms, private personal assistants for housekeeping and laundry, normal pregnancy, and preventive medicine. Extra charge rooms (semi-private or private) and personal assistants for housekeeping and laundry are of special public concern at present. Because hospitalization charges, including nursing, have been kept artificially low, many hospitals have extra charge rooms with an added burden of personal assistants. (Hospitalization charge per day is still only 8,200 yen ($24.60) even for the highest grade of nursing.) Aside from these technical aspects, there are built-in mechanisms for disproportionate increases in health care costs in the future.

High Cost of Medical Technology

First is the advance in medical technology that has particular significance in Japan. Since there is a fierce competition for patients (for example, the advertisement for clinics and small hospitals make up a substantial proportion of the suburban billboards) many institutions also install expensive equipment to attract patients even if insurance reimbursement does not initially cover its cost. This will be aggravated by the tremendous increase of physicians. The number of physicians in 1979 (123.2 per 100,000 population) is projected to reach 180 per 100,000 population by 1990.[14] In 1981 there were already over 2,000 CAT (computerized axial tomography) scanners in Japan.[15] After installation of equipment, there will be every incentive to utilize it as much as possible.

Malpractice suits, though traditionally rare, have been increasing, which may add to the tendency of increased utilization of examinations. It must be remembered that no examination can be considered totally irrelevant for a patient, especially for the elderly.

Difficulties in Planning Health Care Delivery

Second, the system of health care delivery makes planning difficult, particularly in the metropolitan areas. Each clinic or hospital is an independent self-contained organization, competing for patients with its own medical staff. The exchange of personnel or patients would be extremely difficult. Only in some areas, in which the medical resources are geographically and functionally well distributed, can effective planning be realistically conceived.

Aging Population Base

Third is the demographic structure of Japan. The proportion of those over age 65 in the present population of 118 million is 9.0 percent.[16] In the year 2000, the number is expected to grow to 19 million and will compose 14 percent to 15 percent of the population. After the year 2000, it is projected that those over age 65 would increase to an unprecedented level of 18 percent to 20 percent of the population.[17,18] Health care costs of this geriatric population would by itself be a tremendous problem. It is feared that it will be greatly aggravated by the two conditions described earlier. The competition for outpatients and the ready accessibility of health care may have led to a process of early diagnosis and early treatment that has resulted in better health indices. The competition for geriatric inpatients is likely to lead to crushing health care costs that are doubtful to benefit all. Those over age 70 already constitute 24.2 percent of the total population hospitalized. Their average length of stay of 105.1 days is twice the level of the average of the entire population.[19] According to a survey of the entire geriatric population of a community, their current placement status could only be understood from a combination of the subject's disability, the family caring capacity, and the psychological relationship between the subject and the family health care provider.[20] From the importance of the latter factors, it is evident that a new system of evaluating institutional care is needed.

The phenomena of good health indices and the relatively low burden of health care costs in Japan are a result of a complex social history. This chapter has drawn attention only to some aspects that might have relevance to the provision of health care in the United States. These are (1) the historical background in which ambulatory care occupied the dominant position and (2) the health insurance scheme that benefits and intensifies this tendency. These characteristics have been successful up until now in absorbing some of the momentum of the increase in health care costs. However, with the growing proportion of the elderly, a radical new approach in organizing health care is needed.

NOTES

1. Ministry of Health and Welfare, "Health Trend of the Nation," *Kosei-no-shihyo*, 28, no. 9, Supp. (1981): 432–505.
2. Ministry of Health and Welfare (Tokyo: Ministry of Health and Welfare, 1982).
3. C. Nakane, *Japanese Society* (Middlesex, England: Penguin Books, 1973).
4. N. Ikegami, "Growth of Psychiatric Beds in Japan." *Social Science and Medicine* 1-A (1980): 561–571.
5. Ministry of Health and Welfare, *Interpretation of the Point-Fee Tables* (Tokyo: Shakaihoken Kenkyujyo, 1981).
6. Ministry of Health and Welfare, *Report on Social Health Insurance, 1965* (Tokyo: Ministry of Health and Welfare, 1967).
7. Ministry of Health and Welfare, *Report on Social Health Insurance, 1980* (Tokyo: Ministry of Health and Welfare, 1982).
8. S. Fujisaku, "Health Systems and Health Economics," in *Administrative Medicine: An Introductory Manual*, ed. M. Takahashi (Tokyo: Igakusnoin, 1977).
9. Ministry of Health and Welfare, *1957 Patient Survey* (Tokyo: Ministry of Health and Welfare, 1975).
10. Ministry of Health and Welfare, *1979 Patient Survey* (Tokyo: Ministry of Health and Welfare, 1981).

11. Ibid.
12. Ministry of Health and Welfare, *1980 National Health Survey* (Tokyo: Ministry of Health and Welfare, 1982).
13. Ministry of Health and Welfare, *1979 Patient Survey.*
14. "The Need to Respond in Health Economics," *Asahi Seimei,* monthly report no. 149 (Tokyo: Ministry of Health and Welfare, 1981).
15. Ministry of Health and Welfare, *1981 Report from Hospitals* (Tokyo: Ministry of Health and Welfare.
16. Bureau of the Census, *1980 National Census,* vol. 2 (Tokyo: Bureau of the Census, 1982).
17. Institute of Population Problems. *Future Population Problems for Japan—1975–2100 (November 1976 Projections),* research paper no. 213 (Tokyo: Institute of Population Problems, 1976).
18. M. Yasukawa, *Easy Demography* (Tokyo: Japanese Organization for International Cooperation in Family Planning, 1978).
19. Ministry of Health and Welfare, *1979 Patient Survey.*
20. N. Ikegami, "Growth of Psychiatric Beds."

Chapter 4

Hospital Management in Japan: An Overview

JAPANESE AND U.S. HOSPITAL MANAGEMENT PRACTICES

A few facts will bring Japanese hospital management into perspective and serve to differentiate it from practices in the United States. First, the Medical Services Law of Japan, enacted in 1948 under the guidance of the U.S. Supreme Commander for the Allied Forces, defined the responsibilities and requirements of hospitals, their facilities, and personnel. One of these requirements was that the hospital administrator—whose position is a combination of medical director and top administrator—be a physician. This is significantly different from the United States where, with few exceptions, there are no regulations requiring a medical (or for that matter any) degree for a hospital administration post. In Japan a second type of person, who usually has the title "business manager" is often found on the administrative staff. Despite a lack of uniform training and education for hospital management, the position of business manager inevitably involves responsibility for the nonclinical aspects of the hospital.

The next two differences between Japanese and American practices concern the number of hospitals and their ownership. Japan has approximately 9,000 hospitals with 1.3 million beds for its population of 118 million compared to the United States, where there are approximately the same number of beds and 7,000 hospitals for 230 million people. In terms of size almost 80 percent of Japan's hospitals are under 200 beds, and 10 percent are over 400 beds. This distribution differs from the United States, where approximately 50 percent are under 200 beds and about 10 percent are over 400 beds. What is most important is that in Japan there are over 2,000 hospitals with less than 50 beds, and most are privately owned. Indeed, in 1975, of the 7,235 general hospitals, 74 percent were privately owned, frequently by physicians.[1] (These figures refer only to institutions classified as hospitals; they do not include clinics with 19 or fewer beds and with patient stays limited to 48 hours.)

A fourth difference is that, for the most part, physicians who work in hospitals work there full time, while those practicing in clinics tend to stay in that setting full time. In 1980, of the 156,235 physicians in Japan, 77,422 worked full time in hospital practice while 70,393 worked in clinics, without hospital-admitting privileges.[2] Thus, the American concept of attendings with admitting privileges essentially does not exist in Japan.

A fifth difference has to do with average length of stay, which, in Japan, is generally in excess of 30 days. Further refinement of the data, to examine average length of stay for patients over 65, reveals stays in excess of 50 days. This contrasts sharply with the United States, where the average stay is approximately 7 days, with a figure of slightly less than 11 days for patients over 65.[3] Why the great difference? The answer most likely is related to the relative paucity of nursing home beds in Japan: 70,000 there, compared to more than one million in the United States. Thus, the institution that was built and presumably equipped as an acute care hospital, in practice serves as both an acute care hospital and nursing home.

A sixth and final difference occurs in those Japanese hospitals that are not privately owned. This difference is related to the concept that the position of hospital administrator belongs to the senior physician, as a reward for many years of long and faithful service. In a sense then, the hospital administration post is the ultimate recognition of a distinguished career. Further, the hospital administrator may not even be expected to give up clinical medicine; thus the post is also a part-time career.

As a reflection of the role of the physician administrator, hospital administration is taught in about half of the medical schools in Japan as one component of the curriculum. However, postgraduate training for the business manager or the physician who becomes a hospital administrator—or wishes to formally train for hospital administration—is nonexistent in formal academic settings.

HOSPITAL ADMINISTRATION TRAINING

As an illustration of the medical school commitment toward hospital administration education, one can briefly review the hospital and medical administration curriculum at the Keio University School of Medicine. (Keio is considered to be one of the best private medical schools in Japan.) During the four years of medical education the student has a four-and-one-half-hour orientation to hospitals and a tour of the university hospital (during the first term of the second year). In that same term another ten and one-half hours are spent listening to lectures on the role of the hospital in the public health and social systems. These lectures continue during the second term of the second year for another seven and one-half hours. During that second term the medical students also spend twelve hours working on projects at the Keio University Hospital. Finally, during the third year, four and one-half hours are spent studying health law, health economics, and health systems. Additionally, students take related public health and preventive medicine courses. Within the total medical curriculum, less than one percent of the course time is spent studying hospital administration (compared with 15 percent for medicine, 2 percent for dermatology, and 4 percent for psychiatry).

Compared to U.S. medical schools, Keio provides very thorough training in hospital administration; few American schools would devote 39 hours to hospital administration and related courses. However, this may not be an appropriate comparison, because many graduates of Japanese medical schools will eventually work full time in hospitals and play some role in hospital administration.

Other than in medical school, training for hospital administration goes on in a variety of settings, including local or prefectural hospital associations, various professional groups, and the National Institute of Hospital Administration, a government agency founded in 1949. (Originally known as the School of Hospital Administration, the national institute was quite influenced by the work of Mac-Eachern and the Northwestern University hospital administration program.) Since the training at the National Institute of Hospital Administration is the most focused on hospital administration, it is useful to review the 1980 annual report to illustrate the courses offered at this institution.[4] In this report it is noted that eight short courses lasting either eight or nine days were offered: three of these courses were for business managers, two for hospital administrators, two for nursing directors, and one for pharmacy directors. Additionally, a five-day seminar was held on hospital finances, a five-day course on labor relations, a four-day course on hospital architecture, and a three-day seminar on medical auditing. Finally, the institute held two courses, each four months in length, for physician administrators and business managers and a second term-long course for medical records staff. Most attendees were from government hospitals, with a total of 500 attendees for all the institute's courses in 1980. What the other thousands of administrators, nursing administrators, and business managers do for basic and continuing education is not clear.

CASE DESCRIPTIONS

To illustrate the nature of hospitals as well as the practice of hospital administration in Japan, this chapter concludes with short descriptions of three hospitals and one private hospital chain. This will be followed, in the next chapters, with longer case descriptions of three other institutions. The first case in this chapter is an introduction to the corporate-owned hospital; the second looks at a government-owned facility; and the last two examine chain-type operations, one voluntary and one proprietary. These first four cases are presented as an introduction to Japanese hospital management.

Tokyo Private Corporation Hospital

Located a few blocks from a major university hospital, the Tokyo Private Corporation Hospital (a pseudonym) is a 200-bed facility that, from the outside, appears to be another one of the ever increasing Tokyo office buildings. Once inside, the white-uniformed nurses and the characteristic odors signal immediately that this is a medical facility. The hospital is ten years old and provides general medical and surgical services on both an inpatient and outpatient basis to the thousands of employees and their dependents of the Tokyo Private Corporation, the organization that owns the hospital. The hospital is not open to employees of any other work group or members of the adjacent community.

The institution's 200 beds are staffed by 250 persons including 120 registered nurses, 50 business office, clerical, and dietary staff, 50 clinical service (X-ray and laboratory) employees, and 21 full-time medical staff. Augmenting these employees are a number of other persons, who deliver services through outside contractors to perform housekeeping and laundry services, for example. The average length of stay in the hospital is presently 22 days.

The hospital administrator is elected for a two-year term by the other members of the medical staff. After the election the hospital administrator must be approved and appointed by the Tokyo Private Corporation's board of directors. The present administrator has served several terms. The business manager has no hospital management experience and is rotated through the hospital from the corporation's central office.

In the opinion of the hospital administrator, hospitals have a tradition of poor management. Further, he notes that the focus of the hospital should be on "satisfying the needs of the physicians." His conclusion was that a "physician must be in charge and that all decisions should defer to his judgment."

Hospital employees receive the same benefits as other Tokyo Private Corporation personnel. These include twice-yearly bonuses that amount to almost five months' additional salary; twenty days of vacation; and a range of other health and welfare benefits. While quality circles are used in the parent company, they are not found in the hospital. In explaining this, the hospital administrator stated he did not feel that decisions in hospitals lend themselves to participation as they do in industry. Lifetime employment is virtually guaranteed in this hospital, and although the hospital sponsors a variety of social gatherings, the administrator felt there was not much socializing of hospital personnel outside work hours.

As noted at the beginning of this description, the hospital is located only a few blocks from a major university medical center. Despite this proximity, the hospital has its own $1 million CAT scanner, on which it performs an average of eight scans per week. The decision to buy the machine was made by the hospital's executive committee and approved by the parent corporation. Issues of cost implications, reimbursement policies, regulations, and regional planning—all of which give American hospital administrators ulcers—were not significant factors in the decision.

National Medical Center

Located in the Shinjuku section of Tokyo, the National Medical Center is a 1,000-bed hospital owned and operated by the Ministry of Health and Welfare. The origin of this hospital, which now serves as a general medical and surgical facility as well as a research institution, is in the military where, during World War II, the institution served as the First Army Hospital. Although built for 1,000 beds, only 688 beds are operational, and the daily census is approximately 525—for an occupancy rate of almost 76 percent—with an average length of stay slightly under 38 days. Staffing this hospital are 739 personnel including 153 physicians, 346 nurses, and 17 pharmacists.

The facility itself is ten years old, in good repair, with the usual range of high-quality technology to be expected in a regional medical center, including computerized registration and information systems, CAT scanners, and an end-stage renal disease unit. The inpatient facilities, located on 12 floors, are dominated by 2-, 3-, and 6-bed rooms with private rooms on 3 floors. Fifteen nurses are assigned to each 45-bed unit for each 24-hour shift. The hospital maintains an active outpatient service that sees more than 1,200 patients per day. The space is crowded, and there are often long waits for service.

The hospital's director has been in the top administrative position for one year, having previously served as vice director for six years and before that as chief of surgery. His normal workweek is devoted to administration, although he still tries to allocate some time to clinical medicine. According to the director, his main administrative problems revolve around union complaints, and often the issues brought before him are not within his area of authority or responsibility. In analyzing these complaints, he felt that a fundamental problem was that the hospital was too large, resulting in management too far removed from day-to-day activities.

Quality circles do not exist in the hospital; however, there are a number of committees that have been established for the purpose of contributing to the decision-making process. Overall, about ten percent of the staff belong to one or more of these committees, which range in size from 10 to 60 members.

All staff members are civil service employees with life tenure. Despite this there is a 25 percent turnover in the nursing staff due to marriage and relocation; some physician turnover (although no figure could be obtained), with physicians going into private practice or to other hospitals; and a 10 percent turnover of other staff. The hospital sponsors a variety of clubs and social activities and an annual overnight outing for all employees (with smaller groups of approximately 20 percent going on each overnight). The costs for these activities are shared, and participation is high among all groups except the physicians.

The Japanese Red Cross Medical Center

The Japanese Red Cross Medical Center is a modern 880-bed tertiary care facility located in the Hiroo section of Tokyo. It is one of 93 Red Cross hospitals in Japan, and like all the other Red Cross hospitals, its assets—including land, buildings, and capital equipment—are owned by the Red Cross. Despite corporate ownership, this hospital and all the others in the Red Cross chain operate relatively independently, and there are presently no formal regional health services or systems.

With an average length of stay of 24.6 days, the hospital maintains an occupancy rate of 92 percent. Staffing this facility are 1,071 employees, including 109 physicians, 23 pharmacists, and 611 nurses. The outpatient service, as in almost every Japanese hospital, is a busy one, with over 1,700 visits per day. The hospital also maintains a training school for nurses and a residency program for physicians.

The hospital's organizational structure has at its top positions a physician hospital administrator and four physician deputies, who are responsible for the various clinical services. A relatively unique aspect of this hospital's organizational structure is the position of the business manager (whose title is director of administration). Typically business managers handle what can be categorized as the clearly administrative side of the hospital (food service management or the business office, for example). In this hospital the director of administration is also responsible for some of the clinical departments, including nursing, pharmacy, laboratory, and social services. Coordination of this relatively complex organization is the responsibility of two major committees. One of these groups is the policy committee, which focuses on finance, personnel, planning, and outpatient and inpatient affairs. Members of this committee include the hospital administrator, the four physicians who are deputy administrators, and the director of administration and two of his assistants. The second committee, known as the administrative committee, is composed of clinical department heads and focuses on coordinating efforts.

Labor turnover at the hospital is estimated at 20 percent per year and is highest among young physicians looking to use their experience at the Red Cross Medical Center as leverage to obtain a better professional position. Nursing turnover is similar to other institutions, and the reasons are typical: marriage and relocation. In other departments turnover is practically zero, with no staff member having been fired within recent memory.

When the business manager was asked about quality circles, the response was that in a medical facility, quality must be judged by the quality of medical care, and there are numerous activities at the Red Cross Medical Center concerned with assuring quality. Included on their list were periodic outside lectures, death conferences, clinical pathology conferences, and monthly academic meetings.

Staff receive the usual financial bonuses typical of hospitals and industry. However, women who take off the two allowed days per month for their menstrual cycle receive reduced bonuses. Hospital employees can participate in the Red Cross recreational facilities program and utilize the various resorts maintained by the parent organization.

The director of administration of this hospital is particularly interesting in a variety of ways. For him, this is a postretirement position. Prior to joining the Red Cross organization he held a number of government posts, including the director-ship of the social insurance section of the Ministry of Health and Welfare and the directorship of the wage and salary section of the Ministry of Labor. His first postretirement position was with a public corporation responsible for pension plans. Subsequently he joined the Red Cross as its director of personnel and five years ago moved into the hospital position.

Perhaps because of his seniority and record of achievement, the director of administration has been accorded a measure of authority and responsibility unusual for nonphysician administrators. The net result is that the Red Cross Medical Center's approach to nonphysician administration is certainly more typical of an American-style hospital than that of most Japanese hospitals. How well it works in Japan is another matter.

Tokushu–Kai Medical Corporation

To talk of the Tokushu-Kai Medical Corporation is in large measure to speak of the vision of Dr. Torao Tokuda, a 41-year-old surgeon who is the founder and owner of the chain of nine hospitals. The chain, which started with eight hospitals in 1975, is geographically dispersed throughout Japan. According to Tokuda, it is the only private hospital chain so dispersed. In 1982 it was staffed by 2,300 employees, with 3,500 beds functioning at a fifty-seven percent occupancy rate.

All the facilities are modern, and a number of the medical staff, including some hospital directors, were recruited by Tokuda from the United States. The physicians are United States-trained Japanese, but they had been in the United States for so long that their ability to reestablish themselves in Japan was somewhat limited. Part of Tokuda's motivation in developing this system is related to his criticism of Japanese health care. He believes that physicians are too profit oriented and that hospitals are not run in an efficient and effective enough manner. One of his remedies for this situation is to strengthen the position of the business manager; a second crucial element in his organizations is team building.

According to Tokuda, team building goes on in hospitals via continual exchanges of information, including a 15-minute session every day where "morning greetings" are exchanged. This exchange goes far beyond pleasantries: it includes a discussion of the activities of the previous day and the plan for the forthcoming workday. In some hospitals physicians attend these briefings; in others, they do not. Dr. Tokuda notes that hospitals with high physician participation also tend to be better managed. He suggests that "the more people who meet together, the more teamwork that is built."

Tokuda's critics maintain that he is a personal promoter who, although charming, actually operates a chain of hospitals that is on shaky financial grounds because of high costs and low occupancy. These critics note that despite all of Tokuda's speeches, books, and articles his hospitals function similarly to most other private institutions in Japan. To the American observer the Tokushu-Kai chain is an interesting experiment still in its embryonic stage but certainly worthy of careful observation.

REFERENCES

S. Hashimoto and K. Kiikuni, *Health Services in Japan, 1977.* A brochure prepared for the 20th International Hospital Congress (Tokyo, 1977), pp. 7–10.

Prime Minister's Office, *Japan Statistical Yearbook, 1982* (Tokyo, 1982), p. 614.

E. Graves and R. Pokras, "Expected Principal Source of Payment for Hospital Discharges: United States, 1979," *National Center for Health Statistics Advancedata,* no. 75, February 16, 1982, p. 4.

National Institute of Hospital Administration, *Annual Report* (Tokyo, 1980).

Part II

Case Studies and Survey

The next three chapters present case studies of three very different hospitals. The first case examines the workings of an institution owned by a public corporation. Probably the closest analogy in the United States is such independent federal agencies as the Tennessee Valley Authority or the Postal Service. But why look at such a hospital if similar organizations in the United States do not run health care institutions? Basically, there is one reason. In Japan, the government and public corporations are generally thought to represent the best quality institutions and are excellent models of corporate management. Therefore, it became incumbent upon me to examine this type of institution in my search for ideas.

The second hospital studied was a private facility. With the growth of the proprietary sector in the United States, this case study may be particularly interesting to many. However, my reasons for selecting it for this analysis were (1) that it is representative of the most prevalent form of hospital organization in Japan, and (2) from the perspective of the objective of this work, the private hospital offers the opportunity of seeing what goes on when an institution has the flexibility most often found outside of government bureaucracies.

The last hospital considered was St. Luke's, an institution that, because of its history, is an interesting blend of East and West. From St. Luke's we can see what happens when the traditional Japanese approach functions within a hospital that is in many senses American in style.

Each case involved observation, interviews, surveys, and review of written material. As with all case reports, there is a temporal problem. The cases presented here represent the state of affairs in 1982, with limited updating through 1983. Regardless, the cases are meant to illustrate the hospitals' organization and management and give the reader some flavor of these institutions. Finally, some mental gymnastics are required to convert yen to dollars (at the time of the study the conversion rate was approximately 220 yen = $1.00 (U.S.).

Chapter 5

The Public Corporation Hospital

INTRODUCTION

The Public Corporation Hospital is a 30-year-old facility that is an example of those institutions in Japan owned by large corporations, in this case, a public corporation. This hospital is one of 17 owned by the company and is part of an even larger network of health facilities that includes more than 100 health clinics. The hospital, although owned by a public corporation and developed primarily for the use of its employees, accepts patients who are not associated with the company or its related corporations. It is difficult to estimate how many patients are served by the hospital, but as some indicator of its particular population the outpatient clinics maintain 210,000 active files. It is also known that 65 percent of the patients are Public Corporation employees and dependents; 15 percent are employees and dependents of the ministry of which this public corporation was once a part; and 8 percent are persons retired from these two organizations. The remaining patients, who must pay full charges, come from the community or are employed in other organizations. Plans are now being formulated to open the hospital to a wider number of patients covered under national health insurance, which would have the effect of increasing occupancy and perhaps cutting the deficit.

The hospital itself is a 542-bed facility that maintains a 77 percent occupancy rate with an average length of stay, in fiscal year 1981, of 25 days. The staff of approximately 1,000 employees includes 160 physicians, 470 registered nurses, 25 pharmacists, 60 lab technicians, 20 X-ray technicians, 40 system engineers, 34 in food service, 20 in a research institute, 20 in the nursing school, and 150 in the clerical section. The large number of system engineers is explained by the fact that the hospital maintains a complex computer facility that serves as the basis of the hospital's managerial and clinical information systems as well as the research and development arm for the parent corporation's telecommunications applications in the health field.

For the 1,300 outpatients who come to the clinic each day, a visit begins at the registration area. A new patient will have a number of forms to fill out that address the eligibility question and open the necessary patient files. A currently registered patient fills out a check-box-type form and then heads off to his or her clinic of choice. There are no appointment or triage systems, hence each patient selects time, date, and place of visit. The computerized registration system distributes information to the outpatient records room and clinics that a patient is en route. Then, through a system of pneumatic tubes, the records are sent to the appropriate clinic. After completion of the visit the records are kept at the clinic and picked up at the end of the day by a medical records clerk for refiling. In the event that the patient needs some ancillary service or drugs, the patient is given order slips.

Hours after the patient has first arrived, he or she will be ready for checkout at the business office. At that time a final bill for copayments and pharmacy charges will have been prepared. While the X-ray and lab departments respond to service requests without asking for patient prepayment, the final bill must be paid before the pharmacy will dispense its medications to the patient.

PERSONNEL ADMINISTRATION

Almost all the literature on the Japanese approach to management has focused on the personnel administration activities of the large corporation. In the case of the Public Corporation, we have a hospital that is part of one of Japan's largest and most respected public corporations. So the question of how and where personnel administration functions in such a hospital is particularly important.

Organizationally, the personnel manager reports to the business manager, who in return reports to the hospital administrator. The job of personnel manager in this hospital is somewhat circumscribed because many of the hiring decisions are made outside the hospital, by the parent corporation's corporate officials. However, clinically related positions in departments that are doctor run, such as radiology, are filled through the physician department director. The hiring of physicians is a responsibility of the hospital administrator, with the personnel manager as one of four interviewers. Junior-level doctors, although employees of the parent corporation, are essentially outside of the headquarter's jurisdiction. This brings up an interesting problem with residency staff personnel, who essentially have permanent employment status once they begin training. In order to keep training slots open, the hospital director and department heads must provide placement assistance to those completing training; otherwise, the organization could become frozen in its current staffing position.

Staff Turnover

During the course of one year, approximately 90 staff members (9 percent) leave. This will include approximately 12 physicians, 60 nurses, 10 to 12 technicians, and 4 or 5 clerical staff. In the past year only 2 of the 1,000 staff positions were unfilled, and as usual there were no firings. While there is no "lifetime employment" classification, the personnel manager estimates that between 60 and 70 percent of the staff will spend their entire worklife at the hospital. The decision to leave, he noted, was "up to the employee."

Responsible for the institution's administration is a physician who is organizationally designated as the president. His top management team consists of three physician vice presidents, a director of nurses, and the business manager. The ownership of the hospital by the Public Corporation is in evidence in a variety of ways, including the appointment of the president and other top staff as well as the recruitment and placement of administrative and clerical personnel. Thus the personnel department's role is primarily supportive and clerical. For example, it interviews prospective staff, arranges interviews, maintains records, and checks references.

Middle Management Rotation

Of particular interest is the practice of middle managers—such as the finance director or personnel director (or even senior-level staff such as the business manager)—of working at the hospital for three- to four-year tours of duty, having been rotated there from the parent corporation. In a sense the parent corporation treats some aspects of the hospital as it would any of its numerous other activities, and the practice of managers being generalists who can—and should—move through all components of an organization is followed here. As an illustration of this, one can examine the cases of four men who would be considered assistant administrators in an American hospital. Three of the four have worked for the Public Corporation for more than 30 years, and the fourth has been with the company for 22 years. For all of them this was their first job in the hospital, and since it was their first year on the job they are all expected to stay at the hospital for another two or three years. Only one of the four had ever worked in the welfare bureau, that division of the Public Corporation that provides general supervision and direction to the hospital and other health facilities. Incidentally, all four lived in corporation-owned housing.

Staff Evaluation

Staff evaluation is limited to senior-level personnel, such as department directors or deputy directors. In their cases the evaluation occurs on an annual basis, and the results of these evaluations are used in decision making about bonuses and promotions. In the cases of lower level staff being considered for promotion, the opinion of the supervisor weighs very heavily.

In-House Training

Training at the Public Corporation Hospital is handled by individual departments, generally on an on-the-job basis. As is the tradition in Japan, all new employees start at the same time of year, and orientation is a week-long affair. It is an organizationally decentralized program, almost entirely handled by the department where the employee is working.

An employees' suggestion system is also administered by the personnel department and approximately 25 suggestions per year are received. The rewards for these suggestions are book coupons, but in the past two years only 2 of the 50 or so submitted suggestions have been adopted.

Fringe benefits basically correspond to those of other large corporations, including use of the corporation's resort facilities; 20 days per year vacation after one year of service; 7 paid holidays per year; and a liberal sick leave policy. However, when one takes a sick day, a doctor's note must be obtained, and excessive sick leave can result in a diminution of one's bonus. Maternity leave of 12 weeks is also allowed.

Staff Pay Scale

Pay at the Public Corporation Hospital includes a base salary, additional special payments, and a bonus equal to three months' salary. The following list presents the starting base pay for new graduates in a variety of job classifications:

Job Title	Base Salary per Month (in Yen)
Nurse (RN)	117,500
Nurse (LPN)	104,000
Midwife	124,500
Dietician	112,500
Physical therapist	120,600

Occupational therapist	120,600
X-ray technician	115,800
Lab technician	115,800
Dental hygienist	109,800
Physician/dentist	224,800
Pharmacist	128,200

The average annual salary is somewhat higher because of seniority increments and additional payments. For example, a nurse with 8 to 9 years of service will typically earn between 3 and 3.3 million yen per year. A pharmacist with 18 years of service will earn on an annual basis between 5.8 and 6.2 million yen; a clerical staff person with the same years of service will earn from 4.6 to 5 million yen annually. Finally, a resident physician with 3 years of service will earn 4 million yen per year; by the time the physician is a specialist with 10 years of service, the annual salary will be between 7 and 8 million yen, and with 20 years of service it will rise to 9 to 9.5 million yen.

NURSING DEPARTMENT

High-quality nursing is viewed by the Public Corporation Hospital's administration as one of the hospital's major strengths. At the hospital, a nursing director and a staff of ten deputies manage a staff of nearly 500 nurses arranged in a five-level hierarchy, including the nursing director, deputy directors, supervisory nurses, head nurses, and general staff nurses.

Unit-Level Administration

At the unit level nursing administration is delegated to a head nurse. For example, in the case of the 45-bed pediatric unit the head nurse supervises nine staff nurses. The pediatric unit also has, on its staff, a dietician and a bedside teacher who tutors children and is involved in play therapy. All staff participate in formal and informal unit meetings, including listening to shift reports. Housekeeping throughout the hospital has, for the past ten years, been handled on a contractual basis with an outside firm. A slightly contrasting picture at this hospital is presented in the cardiology unit, where there is a total of 42 beds and the normal day shift has five and one-half staff nurses.

At the Public Corporation Hospital the nurses appear to be divided into two groups: the "regulars," that is those who are essentially permanent; and the ones who were called by one supervisor as the "fresh," recent nursing school graduates. The regular nurses, comprising the supervisory and head nurse levels plus some older staff, have spent their entire professional careers at the Public Corporation Hospital. For example, the head pediatric nurse has been at the hospital for 25 years and a head nurse for 10 years; the pediatric supervisor has been at the Public Corporation for 27 years. The latter group, the "fresh" nurses, accounts for almost all the nursing staff turnover. The reasons for this turnover are thought to be marriage, a husband who does not want his wife working, or a young nurse returning to her home prefecture after schooling and a few years of work experience in Tokyo.

Training Programs

Here it should be noted that the Public Corporation maintains its own three-year nursing school, and of the 60 nurses it recruits each year, 50 are from its own graduating class of approximately 85 nurses. The nursing program itself is tuition free, and at the present time the student nurses receive a small stipend of approximately 22,000 yen per month to cover personal expenses.

Supervisory Functions

The job of the supervisory nurses on the medical and pediatric wards is similar to that of any supervisory position, including the functions of scheduling, teaching, patient care, and supervision. On the wards visited, patient care meetings were held weekly, and these meetings were attended by nursing and medical personnel. The nurses interviewed indicated there are a number of small study groups in which three or four nurses, often from the same unit, get together weekly for a two-hour study session followed by dinner.

Much of the after-work socializing among the nursing staff is to be expected since approximately one-third of the nurses live in the nurses' residence, which is adjacent to the hospital. The housing choice is an attractive option for staff: housing in Tokyo is scarce and expensive, and the hospital is located in an active, interesting, and highly accessible part of the city.

Nursing Personnel Management

With a staff of 500 nurses, personnel management of the nursing department is a crucial function. To deal with these issues there is one deputy director of nursing responsible for personnel management and labor relations activities for nurses. According to this deputy director, the major part of her job is assignment of nursing positions to various units and attending several meetings per month with union representatives. Her involvement in wage negotiations is limited since such matters are handled by the Public Corporation at the corporate level. Perhaps her most important concern is morale, which she views as being maintained through "proper job placement, a reasonable volume of work, and the development of a team spirit." Crucial to this is continual staff training, so that nurses "can adequately communicate with physicians."

The volume of work is in large measure defined by the 40-hour workweek, with several hours of overtime per month. Every 12 weeks the nurses rotate to another shift, and they are paid a differential for the evening or night shift.

Team Spirit

Team spirit may be a function of a variety of factors, including attending the same nursing school; living together; and the range of fringe benefits, including social activities, brought together by the employer. According to various nurses there is a fairly high degree of socializing among the younger nurses, but among the older ones socializing is somewhat limited. This is in large part explained by the fact that 38 percent of the nurses are married and are expected to go home after work and tend to family responsibilities. Socializing among nurses also appears to be very hierarchical: senior nurses socialize with other senior nurses, for instance; and are very nursing oriented: physicians for the most part are not included in any social activities. Even on a formal basis it appears that nurses function in a rather limited range. For example, the staff nurses interviewed indicated they only saw the hospital president once a year, at a formal gathering, and they perceived their own career path as being primarily a function of their seniority and the nature of their relationships with their supervisors.

Union Membership

Most of the staff nurses are members of the Public Corporation's medical union, while a minority are members of the Public Corporation's general union. In the past three decades there have not been any strikes, and reports from the staff indicate that serious grievances are few and far between. The union's focus appears to be primarily on wages; work conditions do not appear to be an issue of contention.

Doctor-Nurse Relationship

An important question involves the physicians: How do they relate to the patients and nurses on the wards? The answer is essentially the same as one would get in America. However, to understand this situation we must recognize not only the obvious differences in education and socialization between the doctors and the nurses but also that ward patients stay many times longer than they would in an American hospital. Thus, for many of the patients, the level of services required of the physician on the ward is minimal. And while the physician maintains an office on the ward, the physician's major duties are likely to be in the outpatient areas.

RADIOLOGY DEPARTMENT

In the radiology department, there are relatively clear lines of authority and responsibility between technical and medical staff. The chief of diagnostic radiology, a former member of the faculty of the University of Tokyo Medical School, is in charge of a unit that is staffed by 3 radiology fellows, 2 residents, 3 part-time radiologists, 19 radiology technicians, and 2 clerks. The day-to-day management of the unit is in the hands of the chief radiological technician, who has two deputies, one for diagnostic radiology and one for radioisotope and radiation therapy.

Between 100 to 120 cases per day are seen in the diagnostic radiology unit. Typically, this includes 50 special procedures, such as upper GI series, and 15 CAT scans on the seven-year-old CAT scanner. The technician work force is rather stable, with no workers ever having been fired and only one technician having resigned in the past two years.

Working hours in this unit are the standard 8:30 A.M. to 5:00 P.M., but the staff often meets after work, and many live together in corporation-owned housing and take short vacations together. Continuing education for staff includes several days per year of updating on procedures and equipment. Quality control is primarily maintained by the X-ray technicians, who are responsible for taking and processing their own films. The reasoning behind this is "if there is a foul up the technician must handle it immediately himself." The chief's involvement in such matters is minimal. For the most part technicians are not involved in major departmental decisions such as the purchase of a CAT scanner. A decision of that magnitude is negotiated between the department head and senior administration. The consensus that is developed around that decision will simply not include technical level staff.

The pattern of staff evaluation described earlier is adhered to in radiology. Only senior echelon staff are evaluated on an annual basis. Should a position open up that would involve promoting someone from the lower ranks, this selection would be made on the basis of seniority and a subjective evaluation. In discussions with staff, there were no reservations about this system.

Perhaps the best reflection of the team spirit and attitudes of the nursing and radiology staffs can be observed in the physical environments of the respective departments. In the radiology department, the X-ray technicians share a large room that contains two rows of desks pushed together. The room also has a corner sitting space with couch and chairs, a sink and coffeemaker, and a television. On the television are the various trophies won by X-ray department teams and individuals. In one corner of the room are skis belonging to several members of the department. The sense one gets is of being in a casual shared den or family room rather than bureaucratic office space. As another example, the cardiology nurses have a room where each has a private locker. But in that space there is also a television, plants, coffee pot, cakes, and comfortable seating. It is suggested that the homelike atmosphere created in these various spaces is a reflection of the employees' involvement, commitment, and to a large extent, trust in their organizations. But it should be understood that the physicians share neither physical space nor personal involvement with their technical subordinates in these and likely other departments.

BUSINESS MANAGEMENT

The Business Manager

The senior nonphysician on the hospital's staff holds the title of business manager. Presently the position is filled by a 27-year employee of the parent corporation. For him this is a first experience in a line management position in a hospital. However, because of a previous tour of duty in the Public Corporation's welfare bureau, he is not a neophyte in health affairs. The business manager in this hospital plays a critical liaison role between the parent corporation and the hospital on the issues of finances, personnel management, and labor relations. He is also involved in medical staff matters relating to the appointment of senior physicians since he is usually involved in the interviewing process.

A typical day for the business manager includes any number of meetings with senior administrative and medical staff, parent corporation officials, and representatives of outside organizations such as the various hospital associations. Twice each day the business manager tours the hospital and, as so many of his colleagues in America do, he spends a great deal of his time on countless telephone calls. The critical aspect of the business manager's job, however, is that he is the parent corporation's representative in the hospital and that, after three or four years at the hospital, he will return to a post in the parent corporation.

Medical versus Nonmedical Management Practices

In comparing management in the nonmedical divisions of the parent corporation with management practices in the hospital, the business manager makes some important observations. Uppermost on his list of differences is the fact that in the hospital one has to coordinate the activities of numerous professional groups, each of which not only has pride in its work but a greater orientation to its professional group than the organization. A second major difference relates to the role of women in the hospital organization. In the parent corporation women are not as highly educated as in the hospital, and the parent corporation's staff does not have as high a percentage of women as does the hospital. (At the Public Corporation Hospital 60 percent of the staff are women.)

DISCUSSION

What one observes at the Public Corporation Hospital is a modern, clean, and well-equipped institution. One also sees patients seemingly waiting all over the hospital; by noon, perhaps 150 persons are waiting to have prescriptions filled, and 50 more are waiting in the registration area. In the X-ray department rows of people are also waiting. To the western observer, the number of patients out of bed is particularly striking. Since so much of the care in the Japanese hospital can be classified as intermediate care, this should not be totally unexpected. However, what this does mean is that a significant number of unattended, pajama-clad patients can be seen walking throughout the hospital.

A second aspect of this hospital differentiating it from the typical American hospital is the involvement of family in attending to the needs of patients. For example, family will often do a patient's laundry, prepare snacks, and feed the patient.

Staff Loyalty

Another impression is that of a well-trained and fiercely loyal staff. Nurses and technical staff appear to be committed to spend their entire professional careers at the hospital, and they socialize with one another outside of work. Data from various interviews suggest that nurses are an influential group in this hospital, partially as a result of many having been with the hospital for decades. Indeed, during orientation of the new physicians the nursing director spends an hour and a half with the new doctors, attempting to acquaint them with the idea that nurses are their partners in medical care. The nursing director also warns them to listen to the experienced nurses, especially if they ask the doctor a question in three different ways: "Is this correct?" "Is that what we should do?" and "Is that the exact procedure?" While there is no direct confrontation, there is an accepted convention for calling the activities of the physicians into question.

Fortunately this hospital does not appear to have a problem with physicians, largely because there is an active recruitment program that searches for excellently trained physicians from Japan's best medical schools. This recruitment program follows the traditional Japanese approach of an "old boy–professor" network.

Work Group Stratification

Stratification by work group is also part of life at the Public Corporation Hospital. From talking with the nurses, it is apparent that they do not socialize, on the one hand, with physicians, or on the other, with food service employees. Only senior administrative staff and senior medical staff regularly see the hospital's president, but all employees interviewed felt their supervisors and union presented adequate avenues for communication up the hierarchy. Formal methods of communication include the usual newsletters and weekly bulletins. For management there is also the "ringi" system—essentially a memo routed through the organization for the purpose of having everyone interested in a particular decision advised of the issue and given an opportunity to comment before signing off. Project teams, 13 in all, along with representatives from different departments provide a final mechanism for working together. These teams tackle problems such as balancing the budget, reviewing suggestions, and planning for new categories of patients. Quality circles do not exist in the hospital, although they are used in the parent corporation.

Managerial Generalists

Long hours of work for the administrative staff are typical. Why this is so is unclear. It may be a function of a variety of factors, but one crucial problem is that middle management personnel have no prior experience in health care management. Thus they are expected to learn their job and be productive at the same time. Further aggravating this situation is their brief, three- or four-year tenure on the job. This turnover of senior administrative staff is viewed by some, who voiced a desire for greater managerial stability, as a serious problem. However, the hospital is owned by a parent corporation that apparently shares the prevalent Japanese view concerning the need to have managerial generalists.

Reducing the Deficit

The Public Corporation Hospital is a deficit operation, but because of the parent company's sound financial position the deficit can be absorbed. The cause of the deficit is unclear because of the unavailability of financial data. Steps to reduce the deficit have included exerting greater care over utility utilization, supply inventories, and drugs. Staff reductions in 1983 totaled 42 clerks, nurses, and technicians. Additionally, as noted at the beginning of this case an attempt is being made to raise occupancy by opening the hospital to new patient categories. Perhaps one explanation for the deficit is that, based on comparisons with other Japanese hospitals, the Public Corporation Hospital provides dramatically more and higher quality, unreimbursed nursing service, that is more and better trained nurses, than many other hospitals. If the hospital were to be more responsive to the reimbursement situation in Japan it would replace many of its nurses with lesser trained staff. But the price would be high: the quality of care would decline; it would become more difficult to attract top-flight medical staff; and finally, the institution would no longer be the leading hospital it is now.

Chapter 6

The Kitashinagawa Hospital

One of the most distinguishing features of the Japanese hospital system is the large numbers of hospitals and beds that are owned and operated by private physicians. The Kitashinagawa Hospital, located within a mile of the busy Shinagawa business district in Tokyo, is one of this genre. Kitashinagawa is a residential and commercial area, very crowded and with numerous small businesses and homes, most of the latter being relatively old, since they survived the World War II bombings of Tokyo.

DR. MINORU KOHNO, HOSPITAL FOUNDER

The Kitashinagawa Hospital was founded 30 years ago by Minoru Kohno, M.D., an orthopedic surgeon and former associate professor at one of the earliest of Tokyo's private Western style medical schools. Today the hospital consists of four proprietary facilities, all supervised by Dr. Kohno: Kitashinagawa Hospital number one; Kitashinagawa Hospital number two; Kitashinagawa number three; and Kitashinagawa number five. (In Japan the number four is considered unlucky.) A parent organization, the Kohno Clinical Medicine Research Institute, ties together all of these organizations, plus a hospital drug-and-equipment supply corporation. This case focuses its attention only on the activities of the hospital.

Clearly, the moving force behind the Kitashinagawa Hospital is its rather forceful and charismatic owner. Kohno can be described as both a dreamer of dreams and an implementer of many of those dreams. Not only is he an active, practicing physician, but he is the hospital administrator in title and fact. Kohno's presence is everywhere. For example, two recent newsletters were primarily filled with a speech Kohno made in Korea and a report of a study trip he had taken. One of Minoru Kohno's greatest dreams, and one which he has nursed for 15 years, is the establishment of a medical school in Chiba prefecture. This school, about one hour by car from Tokyo, would admit numbers of students from Japan and selected developing countries. Much of Kohno's seemingly boundless energy is directed at developing this school, which has not yet received its first student, hired its first faculty member, or laid its first brick. Yet the dream persists, and many of Kohno's supporters—and detractors—believe that someday it will be realized.

All four components of the hospital are located within several blocks of one another, with most patients coming from the general neighborhood. The hospital's presence in the area is a function of the size of three of the buildings, which clearly stand out as high-rise structures in a community dominated by one- and two-story houses and shops and the hospital traffic on the streets. Uniformed staff and often, pajama-clad patients, can be seen walking on the streets between the hospital buildings. Another sign of the hospital's presence is its fleet of vans, almost continuously shuttling staff and patients around the area.

FACILITIES

The main hospital, Kitashinagawa Hospital Number Five, is housed in two connected buildings. The older structure, housing 46 beds, was built in 1952, with an unusual twin circular-tower design. The second structure, a conventional rectangular building constructed in 1977, houses 156 beds. The building designated as Kitashinagawa Hospital Number Three houses 139 beds, while Number Two has 120 beds, and number one has 48 beds. Buildings one and three are relatively modern facilities, built within the last decade, while number two is an old building with a dark and dreary atmosphere. The wooden floors of number two are partially covered with linoleum, and the wards are crowded with aged patients, some of whom sleep on mattresses and futons placed on the floor. This building has one main, and rather steep, staircase leading to its second floor. There is some degree of specialization in each of these buildings, with one facility focusing on surgery, one on maternity and ophthalmology, and two primarily specializing in internal medicine.

The older section of the main hospital contains small patient rooms as well as laboratories. The newer section contains patient rooms, operating rooms, radiology, outpatient services, and the range of other supporting activities normally found in a small general medical and surgical hospital. The sense one gets from observing virtually any area of the hospital is that it is a busy and crowded place.

The ground floor of the main hospital is occupied by the registration and outpatient departments and part of the radiology suite, with scores of patients waiting on benches in the main corridor. Patient floors generally have either four-

or nine-bed wards, and during the course of my observations patients were most often in their beds, with nurses frequently at the nursing station and many patients being attended to by privately employed "helpers." In general, the rooms, even the intensive care unit, had beds tightly fitted together. With the exception of an executive health service, all of the areas had this sense of physical closeness and spartan furnishings.

PATIENT VOLUME

The hospital's inpatient occupancy rate averages 93 percent, and the outpatient clinic, which is open on Monday, Tuesday, Wednesday, Friday, and Saturday, sees 150,000 patients a year or approximately 600 a day. The hospital also maintains an emergency ambulance, a new and well-equipped 20 million yen vehicle that is called out ten times per month, as well as an emergency service that records 4,000 visits per year. Outpatient charges average 5,000 yen per visit, while inpatient room charges start at 5,000 yen and go up to 50,000 yen per day. The privately employed helpers charge approximately 8,500 yen per day.

STAFFING

A total of 450 people staff this hospital, exclusive of housekeeping and laundry personnel, who are hired on a contractual basis. Also not included in this figure are the helpers employed as private aides by the patient. Thirty-five full-time and 25 part-time physicians are employed by the hospital. It should be noted that these physicians come from 20 different medical schools, a situation that Dr. Kohno describes as being unusual in Japan and one that, from his perspective, involves breaking down parochial walls as well as the academic clique of a few medical schools.

BUDGET

The total budget for the hospital is three billion thirty million yen. Ninety-five percent of this goes to expenses: 47 percent for salaries and 25 percent for drugs and supplies.

INFORMATION MANAGEMENT

The hospital's information system is tied together with a Digital Equipment 11/70 computer that is programmed in MUMPS. While the computer is heavily used for normal billing functions, it is not evident what patient care functions the computer performs, since patient floors are not equipped with computer terminals. However, since the doctors at the Kitashinagawa Hospital regularly produce a number of professional articles published in the *Bulletin of the Kohno Medical Research Institute* and other journals, it is likely that the computer is used in some clinical investigations.

MANAGERIAL ORGANIZATION

Managing the Kitashinagawa Hospital is Kohno himself, three medical vice presidents, and a treasurer. Over the past several years Kohno has been building a middle management team of *amukadari* (literally, descended from heaven), that is, executives who have had successful careers in other organizations and have now retired and moved into new high-level positions. These new staff serve as top-level consultants along with a 19-member board, which meets three times per year to plan and develop policies for the entire enterprise.

MANAGERIAL PHILOSOPHY

The philosophy of the hospital is deeply rooted in its motto, "Shinryo," which can be translated as either dedicated treatment or true therapy. In a variety of documents, including a pocket-sized green book, the hospital reminds its employees of its motto and the following precepts:

1. We should hold it in our hearts to contribute towards the eternal peace of mankind in the whole world by means of medical science.
2. We should improve ourselves so as to find the greatest pleasure in serving our patients.
3. We should be in constant readiness to sacrifice ourselves and help one another in a spirit of love and harmony.
4. We should strive to cultivate a progressive spirit and always endeavor to develop our ability to the utmost.
5. We should maintain a deep sense of integrity and should always perform our responsibilities with the greatest efforts.

To effect this philosophy, Dr. Kohno asks his staff to provide technically high-quality care delivered with affection, pride, and thoughtfulness. His various mechanisms for arriving at this state include Zen meditation and study tours. Periodically staff are sent on one-week retreats to study and experience Zazen meditation. Kohno's view is that Zazen is a "way of living attentively, joyously, and spontaneously under all circumstances."

Kohno is also a believer in learning from the experiences of others, and he, as well as several hundred of the staff at his hospital, has taken more than 120 study trips. These trips help to identify role models for the Kitashinagawa Hospital and its staff. For example, Dr. Kohno frequently points to the Mayo Clinic as the model for his own hospital as well as his planned medical school.

In some of the literature about Japanese management practices, one reads about such things as company philosophies and songs. The Kitashinagawa Hospital comes closest to matching this model. For example, once per month most of the off-duty staff gather for a Thursday morning meeting in a hall rented at a local bank. This meeting, with over 200 people attending, begins with the singing of the Japanese national anthem, followed by the singing of several of the Kohno Clinic songs. Next, reports are made, and finally an outside speaker makes a presentation.

As another mechanism to effect his philosophy, Dr. Kohno has recently hired a personnel manager who is an expert in the area of employee counseling and conflict resolution. In interviews, Dr. Kohno also points out that his hospital was the first in Japan to set up quality circles, a practice that is now followed in some 80 Japanese hospitals. The Kitashinagawa Hospital's quality circles meet monthly and over the past year have made numerous suggestions that have saved the hospital money. This, Kohno notes, is an example of his "bottom up" approach to management. In the next two sections we will briefly look at how the radiology and nursing departments reflect the Kohno approach to management.

RADIOLOGY DEPARTMENT

Eleven technicians are the primary staff responsible for the five-room radiology operation at the Kitashinagawa Hospital. The hospital does not employ a full-time radiologist, depending instead on the services of a part-time radiologist who comes in twice a week.

A typical day's activity in radiology will include taking 80 flat plates, 13 CAT head and 8 CAT whole body procedures. In general, patients do not wait more than 20 minutes for the procedures, and according to the chief technician, complaints are rare. As is customary in most Japanese hospitals, the X-rays are read by the physician ordering the procedure.

Staff leadership is in the hands of the chief technician, who has worked at the hospital for 26 years. Meetings are held three times each week beginning at the end of the normal work shift and typically last until 6:00 P.M. or 6:30 P.M. Two of these weekly meetings focus on professional issues, usually related to radiology techniques and equipment, while the third meeting has as its objective building better relations and communications among staff. The chief's continuing education is also supplemented with three courses outside the hospital each year. As is typical throughout the hospital, the radiology staff appeared very loyal to the institution and usually attended the monthly Thursday meetings, participated in hospital extracurricular activities, and frequently used the hospital-owned resort areas for vacations.

NURSING DEPARTMENT

Of the 450 employees at the hospital, 265 are in the nursing department: 230 are registered nurses and 35 are assistant nurses (the equivalent of licensed practical nurses). Managing this group is a chief nurse, 12 associate chief nurses, and 21 head nurses. Meetings of the senior staff to discuss policy and management issues are held several times each month, and 15-minute briefing meetings are held daily.

The nursing staff is evaluated on a semiannual basis. Data collected from this evaluation are reviewed by the senior nurses and used in promotion and bonus deliberations but not shared with the nurse who has been evaluated.

Turnover of staff is an important issue in the nursing department, with 40 to 50 nurses leaving each year. Thirty to thirty-five percent of the nurses are married, and according to the chief nurse the major reason for resignation is to have children. A second significant reason for resigning is that many of the nurses are returning to school to earn a bachelor's degree.

Of the nursing staff, approximately 35 percent have worked at the hospital for more than five years. The supervisory-level nurses all have at least ten years of nursing experience and supervise 12 to 18 nurses. Perhaps because of their seniority and positions, the supervisory nurses' socializing with other staff is limited. However, a number noted that when they were younger they were active in a range of activities including sports, flower arranging, and tea ceremony clubs.

PERSONNEL

As noted earlier, the hospital has recently hired a personnel manager, who is responsible for staff counseling and conflict resolution. In this nonunionized hospital the role of personnel would appear to be critical, particularly since Dr.

Kohno's ideas and ideals play such an important role in the personnel management tone within the organization.

Reflections of management's attitude toward personnel can be seen in a variety of areas, in particular, salaries and fringe benefits. While a total salary schedule was not available for review, it was discerned that the following starting salaries exist at the Kitashinagawa Hospital:

Title	Annual Salary (in Yen)
Nurse (RN)	160,000
X-ray technician	130,000
Clerk	120,000
Physician	300,000

In addition to the basic salary, male employees receive a 1400Y monthly allowance for a wife, plus a 1300Y per month allowance for each child. The hospital provides a daily lunch to employees at a cost of 150Y per day; the cost of the meal is actually 350Y. Employees can also receive a home purchasing loan from the hospital equal to eleven months' pay. Finally, the hospital provides a range of sports teams, resorts, and clubs. Partial payment for these benefits is paid by a two percent monthly deduction from the base salary; the hospital pays the additional costs. The hospital allows for 20 vacation days per year, and employees work 35 hours a week; five days a week. While women are entitled to six weeks of maternity leave, they are not allowed days off during their menstrual time.

DISCUSSION

It is difficult to generalize from the limited experience of one institution. But if Kitashinagawa Hospital is any reflection of its genre (the proprietary Japanese hospital), the class has some important strengths and weaknesses. The weaknesses are that the hospital, in order to earn a respectable return on its investment, must maintain minimal staffing levels and build facilities with no excess space. Further, investments in facility maintenance must be evaluated very carefully, always balancing potential short- and long-term expenses and revenues.

Staffing Ratios; Condition of Facilities

One might argue that staffing ratios at Kitashinagawa are lower than at the other hospitals studied because of its patient mix and staff efficiency or because the two other hospitals studied had teaching programs. Whether these differences alone can account for the difference is difficult to say. However, it is clear that the facilities of the Kitashinagawa Hospital were, considering their age, in less satisfactory shape than the facilities at a number of other Japanese hospitals. Whether this is due to the initial quality of construction or maintenance, again, is hard to say. However, under the current reimbursement system—which does not provide for reimbursement for new construction or depreciation—and in which procedures are paid for at the same rate regardless of the hospital or the quality of its staff and physical facilities—the incentive is certainly limited to both invest in new buildings and go beyond minimally acceptable staffing levels.

The Leadership of Dr. Kohno

On the positive side, the hospital does offer an excellent view of the impact of strong leadership. In Japanese hospital and medical circles, Dr. Kohno is viewed as an important, albeit controversial, person. Through the force of his charismatic personality and strong political sense, he has been able to build a multifacility hospital and assorted other organizations that both deliver patient care and make a profit. Patients, who clearly have other choices if they are willing to leave the neighboring area, apparently are satisfied enough to flock to the outpatient clinic and hospital, despite what appear to western eyes as barely minimal facilities.

One must be impressed with Dr. Kohno, a single person who can exert such influence over the direction of an entire organization. Taking Kohno at his word, he has introduced into his organization many of those aspects of management that American managers have become so enamored of, including monthly meetings; song singing; Zen meditation; shared traditions, such as study trips, resorts, teams, and clubs; a five-day work week; quality circles; and most recently, a human relations counselor.

Looking Toward the Future

Finally, one must wonder about the vulnerability of the Kitashinagawa Hospital, since it is built so exclusively around the personality of Kohno. In recognizing this, Kohno has started to develop a new top management team that presumably will guard the legacy into the twenty-first century. Whether the spirit can continue without the man will thus be the next major challenge to face the Kitashinagawa Hospital.

Chapter 7

St. Luke's International Hospital

To Americans, St. Luke's International Hospital is perhaps the most interesting of Japanese hospitals because it approximates the American approach to delivering hospital-based care while simultaneously retaining many of the traditional Japanese approaches to managing staff.

St. Luke's is located in the Tsukiji section of Tokyo, best known as a wholesale fish and grocery marketplace teeming with people almost around the clock. Only a few minutes walk from the Ginza, the area has a mixture of buildings, stores, and residences, particularly, large apartment houses. The hospital itself is in one of those unique physical locations that has a daytime population dramatically higher than its evening population. The latest statistics indicate there is a daytime population of 780,000 people in Chou ward (at a radius of approximately two kilometers from the hospital) and a nighttime population of 93,000. The area is also heavily populated on weekends since the five-and-one-half- or six-day work-week is not unusual in Japan, and stores in the Ginza area are normally open on Sunday. Present forecasts indicate that the areas adjacent to the hospital will continue to grow, and even a casual stroll demonstrates that large buildings are going up on vacant sites. If, as discussions indicate, the wholesale fish and grocery marketplace is relocated, this area could be in for a major building boom.

The hospital owns three economically valuable blocks in Tsukiji. One block borders the river and contains a nurses' dormitory and several other small buildings. A second block has a number of low-rise, barracks-type buildings, some of which are over 50 years old. The third block houses the hospital and the St. Luke's College of Nursing.

HISTORY

St. Luke's has an interesting and important history, which begins in 1900, with the American Rudolf Teusler, M.D., being sent to Japan by the Episcopal Medical

Mission. By the time of Teusler's death, in 1934, the foundation of what is today St. Luke's was well in place. During his lifetime, St. Luke's occupied four different physical plants, the last one, opened in 1934, comprising most of the hospital's present physical facility.

Teusler began with a small dispensary and ten beds. In the ensuing years prominent physicians became affiliated with St. Luke's, and it became the major hospital used by the foreign community in Tokyo. During World War II, St. Luke's was not damaged, and after the war it was taken over by the occupation government as the main U.S. Army hospital in Tokyo. At the time of the takeover the facility was only 11 years old, not damaged by the war, and had the feel, in terms of space, architecture, and equipment, of an American hospital. Even today, entering the main lobby and walking toward the chapel would give many an American a sense of déjà vu—for me, this hospital with its dark wood paneling and terrazzo floors was strongly reminiscent of the Presbyterian Hospital of New York.

Eleven years after the takeover, the United States government turned the hospital back to the St. Luke's staff, who in the interim had labored in a 25-bed hospital with an outpatient clinic that saw over 600 patients per day. From most accounts the hospital's plant was under considerable stress during the occupation, particularly in the early 1950s when St. Luke's was used as a 1,000-bed hospital for casualties of the Korean War. Capital improvements by the U.S. government during this period were limited so, in 1956, the St. Luke's staff inherited a much used facility.

In the 1960s a new outpatient wing was added, and in the 1970s serious consideration was given to adding a $25 million wing, which would house 12 new operating rooms, a new laboratory, a new radiology facility, and 90 private beds. This plan was not implemented because of the cost and the desire to eventually build an entirely new replacement facility for the old hospital, a project that is now in the functional planning stage.

At present, St. Luke's is a 341-bed hospital, with 7,455 admissions per year. It has an average length of stay of 13.4 days and a two-month waiting list for elective surgery and its preventive health checkup program (known as the "human dry dock"). The hospital's 15 clinical divisions see 1,384 outpatients each day, 63 of whom are new patients.

HOSPITAL ORGANIZATION

The hospital's organization chart is quite similar to that of an American voluntary hospital, with a 15-member board of trustees delegating authority and responsibility to a hospital administrator, who also serves as the hospital's medical director. In addition to this person, there are two physicians who carry vice-director titles and serve as senior administrators for the clinical departments. The business administration aspects of the hospital are the responsibility of the business manager, who is assisted by a number of senior-level staff. The board meets four times each year to review, comment, and approve major changes such as the purchase of major capital equipment. The board also appoints a long-range planning committee, made up of senior-level staff plus several board-appointed outsiders, which meets once a week and discusses hospital finances and operations.

The present hospital administrator (and medical director) is a senior physician who was elected by his medical staff colleagues. He will serve in this post until he reaches the mandatory retirement age of 65. Other top management staff include the two previously noted vice-directors, the director of nursing, and the business manager. A crucial policy and planning role is played by the steering committee of the hospital, which consists of the director, two vice-directors, business manager, director of nursing, chief of finance, and the personnel manager, who serves as the secretary of the committee. Once a week, on Tuesday mornings, from 8:15 A.M. to 9:00 A.M., this group meets to address important issues, such as the purchasing of new equipment costing up to one million yen (purchases over this amount require board approval). It appears that this committee has perhaps the most crucial role in charting the hospital's future.

FINANCE

Income

The hospital's operating budget is approximately 5.5 billion yen, with over 90 percent generated from patient and patient-related revenues. The inpatient income of 3 billion yen and outpatient income of 1.7 billion yen include the fees received from the various health insurance programs, patient copayments, and supplemental charges for private rooms. Approximately 20 percent of the income is derived from pharmacy charges, which is significantly lower than the 30 to 35 percent pharmacy income typically found in Japanese hospitals. One component of the operating income is the 9 million yen derived from tuition fees obtained from students in the hospital's two-year registered nurse (RN) program. The RN program trains practical nurses for the RN licensure; presently, 30 students per year are accepted into the program. This two-year diploma program is separate from the four-year baccalaureate program, which is the responsibility of the administratively independent St. Luke's College of Nursing.

The hospital's nonoperating revenue of 467 million yen comes from interest on endowment; interest on patients' deposits (upon admission each patient is required to make a 100,000 yen deposit against the copayment expenses); and income from the "human dry dock" program (preventive health physicals). The hospital also receives a 22 million yen subsidy from the Japanese government for its medical and nursing education programs.

Expenses

The largest single expense category is for personnel-related expenses, and depending on what is placed in that category the figure can range from 52 to 54 percent of the total expenditures. Medically related expenses, which include pharmaceuticals, food, laboratory supplies, and radiological supplies, represent 26 percent of the expenditures. Of particular note in the other expense categories is the 11.8 million yen the hospital allows for bad debts and patients who cannot pay insurance deductibles. This category accounts for .002 percent of the budget. A second category of particular interest is the 81.7 million yen in real estate taxes the hospital is obligated to pay to the prefectural government. St. Luke's is what Americans would classify as a nonprofit hospital; thus in the United States it would be exempt from federal, state, and local taxes. In Japan there is an exemption from national, but not local, taxes—in this case the tax amounts to 1.6 percent of the hospital's operating income.

The assets of the hospital are approximately 3.3 billion yen, with liabilities of approximately 1.7 billion yen and equity of 1.3 billion yen. Much of the equity is tied up in endowment funds that are used for staff enrichment and improvements to the hospital's physical plant.

The hospital's financial picture for the past 20 years has been mixed, with the "profit and loss" statement showing a deficit for every year from 1959 until 1981 when, for the first time in over two decades, a modest profit (161 million yen) was attained.

NURSING

As at most American hospitals, nursing is the largest single department at St. Luke's, in terms of staff, with 267 nurses, all of whom are RNs except for one practical nurse. Of these nurses, 60 percent graduated from St. Luke's College of Nursing or the hospital's own nursing school.

Department Organization

The nursing department is headed by a director of nursing, who is a graduate of St. Luke's College of Nursing and a veteran of 27 years with the hospital. Second in command is a vice-director, who is assisted in the management of the nursing staff by 13 supervisors and 14 head nurses. Once per week this senior staff meets formally to discuss major issues and problems. One member of this group described these sessions as "hot discussions." Examples of recent issues considered include nursing standards, clinical procedures, and the coordination of nursing activities with those of other departments.

In addition to the weekly formal meeting there is a daily 15-minute conference, where management is briefed on items of current significance. On one Tuesday the 15-minute meeting lasted 35 minutes, while the nurses discussed plans for an upcoming fire drill. On the nursing units there is a 15-minute daily conference during the middle of the day shift. Typically this meeting is held from 1:45 P.M. to 2:00 P.M. and focuses on updating the staff on current issues as well as reviewing the status of the unit's patients.

Continuing Education

Continuing education is a major activity of the nursing department at St. Luke's. Perhaps because almost every nurse at the hospital is an RN and most hold a baccalaureate degree, there is intellectual pressure for continuing education as well as a desire on the hospital's part to promote such activity. Further, the continuing education program is viewed by nursing and administration as a cornerstone of the hospital's recruitment and retention policies.

Continuing education for nurses can be viewed as beginning with a student's training at either the hospital's or college's nursing program; in both instances the need for continual professional education is stressed. Since many of St. Luke's nurses come from these programs, there is already a cadre of nurses socialized to the importance of continuing education.

After hiring, new nurses are introduced to the hospital with the four-day general hospital orientation (which is discussed in detail later in the chapter) plus a six-day nursing orientation. Further, a weekly hour-and-one-half follow-up orientation is held for new nurses for their first three months on staff.

Other aspects of the continuing education program are journal clubs, joint conferences with physicians to discuss new techniques, and a range of specialty courses including those in intensive care nursing, cardiac care nursing, and leadership. Most activities are scheduled so that nurses on the various shifts can take advantage of them but, as at most institutions, the majority of nurses are on the day shift, and so much of the informal teaching goes on during that time. However, with only 6.7 percent of the nurses married, a figure somewhat lower than at the other hospitals studied, and 45 percent living in the nearby dormitory, participation in the continuing education programs is not a problem. Thus the theoretical 40-hour workweek may be an understatement if off-duty participation in hospital activities is included in this figure. Approximately 10 percent of the nurses also enroll in educational courses outside of the hospital but usually in the Tokyo region and at their own expense.

Turnover

Despite competitive starting salaries, available free housing, a first-rate continuing education program, and the prestige of an institution with an international reputation, turnover of the nursing staff is a significant issue at St. Luke's. In 1970 turnover was as high as 47 percent, but since the mid 1970s the rate has hovered around 30 percent. This figure, while considered acceptable in the United States, is considerably higher than the general labor turnover in Japan; much higher than the typical turnover rate of hospital workers (other than nurses) of 5 percent; and somewhat higher than the usual nurse turnover rate in Japan of 25 percent. The explanation for this level of turnover appears to be that most St. Luke's nurses are recruited directly from the hospital's own nursing programs, and a significant percentage of these women are not from the Tokyo area. For example, in the class that began the hospital program in 1982, only 1 of the 30 students was from Tokyo; 3 others were from the region; and the other 26 lived a considerable distance from the Tokyo area. While some leave for more attractive positions in the Tokyo area, many follow the traditional pattern of working at the hospital for several years before returning to their home prefecture to marry and raise a family.

Retention and Recruitment

Turnover of the nursing staff is an important issue at St. Luke's since the vast majority of time and resources involved with staff recruitment is focused on nursing. The hospital, in the last few years, has begun what might be called a long-range marketing program, which involves maintaining contact with other nursing schools and placing advertisements in a bimonthly controlled-circulation nursing magazine that is distributed to recent nursing school graduates.

The problem of recruitment and retention may become more serious in the near future when Toranomon Hospital, a highly regarded government facility, completes its expansion from 600 to 1,000 beds in April 1984. This hospital, located only a few kilometers from St. Luke's, may attract a large number of recent St.

Luke's graduates—or even present staff members—because of a newer facility and competitive salaries.

St. Luke's also labors under the disadvantage of having a very small number of nurses with long tenure. Only 1.1 percent of the nurses have been at St. Luke's for more than 30 years; 3.0 percent for more than 20 years; 4.5 percent for more than 10 years and 10.4 percent for more than 5 years. In the next few years, the basic strategy of nurse retention, that is, a fair salary and benefits, good working conditions, and a first-rate continuing education program will be under its most severe test.

Staff Evaluation

Evaluation of the nursing staff takes place twice each year. These formal evaluations look at a variety of categories including punctuality, attitude toward self-development, courtesy, attitude, competence, and productivity. Evaluation data are reviewed by the nurse supervisor, but there is no direct feedback to the nurse unless there are substantial problems. In such cases the nurse supervisor (or the personnel manager) will meet with the nurse. Indirect feedback comes by way of the bonus payment, which is awarded to each staff member twice per year.

In general, complaints about the nurses are limited to minor issues such as the problem of new staff who do not know how to present their reports accurately or an occasional criticism about the amount of time nurses spend charting at the nursing stations. Nurses, on the other hand, complain about the old facilities and equipment and that they are called upon, albeit not too often, to do housekeeping and laundry chores for patients. Nurses sometimes perform these chores because St. Luke's, unlike many hospitals in Japan, does not allow the patients to personally employ personal service aides.

The Pediatrics Ward

While there is no such thing as a "typical time" on a "typical" floor at St. Luke's—or at any other hospital—one can certainly catch the flavor of life for the nurses by observing activities on a patient floor, in this case, pediatrics. Pediatrics is a 51-bed unit; 35 patients were there on the day I visited. In addition to the eight nurses working on the unit, there was one housekeeper (a contract employee), one secretary, two nurses' aides, and one teacher. According to the supervising nurse who maintained her desk at the nurses station, which is located in the middle of the floor, half of the children on the unit had some form of cancer. This is largely a function of the hospital having on its staff a world-renowned hematologist, who maintains his component transfusion unit on pediatrics; many of the cases on pediatrics are under his care.

Physically, the pediatric unit is T-shaped with several large wards and a few semiprivate rooms, a newborn nursery, several isolation rooms, a combination playroom/classroom, and a kitchen with microwave oven, refrigerator, and other equipment usually found in a typical American hospital's nutrition unit at a nursing station.

The nursing station appears to be in the middle of a corridor. Actually it consists of several desks and chart racks positioned in front of a large room, which opens onto an indoor balcony that overlooks the interior of a five-story gothic chapel. Each floor is set up similarly, so that patients can attend church services without leaving their floor. The room behind the nursing station also holds an assortment of items including books, tables, a coffee pot, and a television. Although it is not usually used by more than one or two people, it is a space where small meetings can be held. In a private room off to one side of this space the residents have their offices.

Based on my limited observations, the nursing unit is a busy place. For example, during a half-hour period in which I kept a record of telephone usage, there were ten incoming phone calls and two outgoing calls. Pediatric residents were in evidence as they walked past the nursing station on their way to treatment rooms. Medication carts rattled by. A medical photographer came on the unit. Parents walked by; messengers were seen coming and going, delivering a wide range of supplies. The sense is of a busy but organized place. It was clear that there was a physician present on the unit, and that most of the nurses were busy with patients, not paper. At one point a young resident went to fetch a boy in order to administer his treatment. As they walked by, en route to the treatment room, the tension could be seen in the boy's face; nevertheless he walked along gamely, hand in hand with the resident. A few minutes later they came by again, still holding hands, but a more relaxed and talkative boy was heading back to his room with his new friend, the doctor.

Daily Staff Meeting

On pediatrics, 1:45 P.M. to 2:00 P.M. is reserved for the daily nursing staff meeting. Despite the official tone of the meeting and the alleged Japanese penchant for orderliness, not everyone is at the meeting or even on time. Presiding at the meeting is the head nurse, a 1976 graduate of St. Luke's College of Nursing who has been a head nurse for three years. The meeting also involves all on-duty nonmedical staff, including the aides, teacher, and secretary. However, the only talking done is by the nurses; for the most part the conversation is dominated by the head nurse and the supervisor. The supervisor is also a St. Luke's graduate who, although she has worked at the hospital for only three years, graduated from St.

Luke's 18 years ago and then, for family reasons, went to work in a neighboring prefecture.

The picture one is presented with is that of an active and colorful ward with nurses, most of whom are young, busily dispensing medications, taking children to the toilet, chasing after kids, and responding to a variety of demands. What was not observed on pediatrics—or on any other unit—were nurses or other staff engaged in social discussions or simply relaxing. However, it was not unusual to see at least one, and sometimes two or three, nurses at the station involved in charting activities. Since almost all aspects of medical records are done by hand at St. Luke's (including physician's summary statements), the fact that nurses spend so much time charting is not surprising.

RADIOLOGY

Radiology is a service that most patients experience but know little about. At the St. Luke's radiology department, approximately 150 examinations are performed each day, about a third of these are prescheduled. On average, ten whole body CAT scans and ten head CAT scans are also performed each day. Nonscheduled patients usually have to wait, sometimes more than an hour, and this is a primary source of complaints. The physical facilities of the radiology department do nothing to alleviate this problem since space is tight and the waiting room is the corridor, thus precluding any patient privacy.

Staffing the diagnostic radiology section are 2 full-time physicians, 3 full-time radiology residents, and 2 part-time radiologists. Assisting them are 20 technicians, 3 transcribers, 3 clerks, and 5 nurses permanently assigned to the department.

Requesting Physician and Radiologist Read X-Ray

Perhaps of greatest interest and importance is that at St. Luke's every X-ray is read by a radiologist, and both a report and the X-ray itself are returned to the physician who requested the radiological examination. This reporting process, relatively rare in Japan and the United States, is carried through in order to provide a quality control check for radiology as well as to educate the physicians. In Japan there are only 1,500 fully trained radiologists and another 1,500 physicians with a strong enough interest in the field to join the Radiology Society of Japan. The reimbursement system pays the care provider the same amount regardless of who reads the X-ray, radiologist or primary care physician, and only one fee is paid per film or procedure. Thus, what one sees is hospitals taking a large number of films, with the reading left to the physician who ordered them or perhaps to a part-time radiologist who comes in once or twice weekly. One can only wonder what goes on in the 2,300 hospitals with CAT scanners!

Continuing Education

Continuing education in the radiology department is essentially segregated by work group. The doctors have weekly conferences among themselves and often go to other hospitals, medical schools, or meetings of professional organizations for conferences. The technicians have twice-monthly conferences, the clerks meet weekly, and the continuing education of the nurses comes under the purview of the nursing department. The major intergroup professional conferences occur when a new technique is being initiated.

Socializing among the entire radiology staff is limited to a once-a-year retreat to the Hakone Mountain–area hot springs and to quarterly parties. The radiologist in charge of the diagnostic section typically goes out once per month to "drink some sake with the technicians."

PERSONNEL

Perhaps the basic attitude toward personnel relations at St. Luke's was best reflected by one supervisor who, in response to my question about firing an employee, noted that "firing is very painful because it reflects on the manager as well as the employee."

The role of the personnel department at St. Luke's is similar to that of personnel departments in Japanese industry as reported in the literature. According to the hospital's personnel manager, it is also similar to that of numerous other Japanese hospitals.

Recruitment and Hiring

A crucial function of the personnel department is the recruitment and hiring of staff. In 1982, 87 new staff were hired. The distribution of the new hires was as follows:

Job Title	Number
Nurses	70
Lab technicians	6
X-ray technicians	2

Dieticians	2
Pharmacist	1
Clerks	2
Medical records librarians	4

For the dietician, pharmacist, and medical records positions, no advertising was placed since personnel with the appropriate qualifications were readily available. Advertisements and contacts with professional schools led to 80 nurse applicants (60 from the two St. Luke's programs—essentially the entire graduating classes); 20 applicants for the lab technician jobs; 5 applicants for the X-ray technician jobs; and 50 applicants for the clerical positions, which were advertised in the local daily newspaper.

Applicants are given a one-hour examination that measures their technical skills. These exams were developed by the hospital over the years and are used in virtually every job category. Passing applicants are then interviewed by the personnel manager and the appropriate department head. Hiring decisions are made by a consensus of those involved in reviewing the applicants. Interviews are usually 20 to 30 minutes long, and after the interviews references are normally checked by telephone or mail, although some skepticism was evident as to the value of these references.

Personnel Evaluations

A second crucial function of the personnel department is the review of the annual evaluations and determination of the bonus compensation. Personnel gets involved in the review process when a staff member has a particularly poor evaluation. In such cases either the personnel manager or an assistant will meet with the staff member for counseling. The calculation of the bonus, about which more is presented in a subsequent section, is fairly straightforward for most staff, since the bonus percentage figure is negotiated with the union and varies little from year to year. Extra bonus payments are awarded to staff who have better-than-average evaluations, and the personnel department is responsible for calculating ratings and then figuring bonuses for all staff.

Union Negotiation

Wage (including bonus) negotiation is a third important personnel function. St. Luke's has two unions: one with six members, which is affiliated with a national radical union and the second with several hundred members, which is a union of only St. Luke's Hospital staff members—from an American perspective it would be considered a company union. Personnel's responsibility is to negotiate wage rates and administer the grievance mechanism. (In 1981 there were less than 15 filed grievances, dealing primarily with minor issues.)

A final role for personnel is in staff orientation. All new staff begin in April, as is customary in Japan, and the personnel department plans and runs an extensive four-day program that every new staff member, except physicians, attends; perhaps this is a reflection of the physicians' special status.

Of particular interest is St. Luke's salary structure and orientation program; in the following sections they will be reviewed in some detail.

Salary Structure

In addition to a monthly salary, the typical employee receives an additional 30 to 40 percent payment for allowances plus a range of fringe benefits. The official workweek is planned as a 7½-hour workday five days per week and an additional 6-hour workday once in every two-week period. Starting monthly base salaries for staff are as follows:

Title	Monthly Salary (in yen)
Clerk (recent H.S. grad)	109,000
Clerk (recent college grad)	121,000
Pharmacist	126,000
Laboratory tech. (3 yrs. coll.)	125,000
Laboratory tech. (4 yrs. coll.)	127,000
X-ray technician	127,000
Nurse (diploma, RN grad)	135,000
Nurse (B.S.)	138,000
M.D. (just graduated)	167,000
M.D. (2nd year)	232,000
M.D. (3rd year)	257,000

In general these salary differentials are related to educational levels, although it is clear that the additional years of training for a physician pay off to a greater extent than additional years in other professions. There is no dispute with the union over these differentials.

Bonus Awards

In addition to the basic monthly pay, employees receive these monthly payments: a 6000Y bonus if not absent during the month; a 15,000Y inflation bonus; a 14,500Y housing allowance if married, 7000Y allowance if single; and a 3000Y allowance per child. Twice a year, in June and December, each staff member gets a bonus payment. In 1982 this equaled 2.07 times the base salary for the June bonus and 3.03 times the base salary for the December bonus. Individuals whose evaluations are above average for their departments receive additional bonuses amounting to a maximum of 50,000Y for nonphysicians and 100,000Y for physicians. Bonuses are given to all staff, including those whose performance has been less than satisfactory. Over the last five years the bonus multipliers have remained fairly constant.

Pension System and Lump Sum Payment

All hospital staff with more than one year and one day of service are entitled to *taishokukin*, that is, a lump sum payment when they leave, either through retirement or resignation. After one year employees are entitled to .6 of one month's salary. After two years the multiplier becomes 1.2; after three years, 1.8; after four years, 3.2; and after five years, 4.4. Thereafter the multiplier is the number of years' service. Thus a physician retiring at the mandatory retirement age of 65 will receive, assuming 30 years of service, a lump sum payment of 30 times the monthly base salary. St. Luke's also maintains its own pension plan, which pays approximately 30 percent of the base salary to any employee who retires with more than 25 years of service. The government's pension plan also pays approximately 40 to 45 percent of the base salary. It is estimated that a retired staff member will normally receive, in pensions, approximately 65 to 70 percent of his or her base salary, plus a sizable lump sum payment. The retirement age at the hospital varies: it is 65 for physicians; 60 for nurses; and 55 for other staff who are high school graduates. If an employee works for St. Luke's for more than 25 years but leaves before retirement, the pension is lost but the lump sum payment is awarded.

Other benefits administered by personnel include resorts where staff can rent accommodations at very modest prices; a range of club activities; free housing for nurses; and some limited housing for other staff. Discount meals are also provided; for example, 100 yen buys a box lunch of tempura-fried shrimp and other fish, rice, a few vegetables, and soup.

Orientation

A very important function of the personnel department is directing orientation. A review of the 1982 orientation schedule provides a sense of the investment that the hospital makes in this activity. The first sessions were held on Saturday and opened with the hospital director's hour and a half presentation on the history of St. Luke's. Following this, the business manager gave a half-hour talk on the organization and management of the hospital. Next, the director of nursing and the chaplain gave half-hour talks. After lunch, the personnel manager and his staff used two and a half hours to discuss salaries, taxes, fringe benefits, and work regulations.

Monday, the second day of orientation, began with the new employees introducing themselves. The next two hours were devoted to a journal club discussion of a short book that all new staff had previously received and were expected to read. (The book is about the history of St. Luke's and its founder, Dr. Teusler, and his philosophy.) The afternoon was devoted to discussions about the attitudes of personnel to one another and to patients, plus a presentation on fire safety and security.

The third day began with an overview of the hospital's administration followed by instruction and role playing on telephone usage. After lunch the new staff were taken on a two-hour guided tour of the hospital, followed by discussions on attitude and courtesy.

The last day of orientation began with more discussions about attitudes, followed by a presentation about the employee health service. Lunch on this final day was a special event, with employees going to lunch with their new supervisor. Following this meal, a distinguished person from outside the hospital was brought in to present a closing lecture.

Staff Communication

Communication is viewed as crucial to successful personnel management at St. Luke's. As noted earlier, there is a range of extracurricular activities financed by a small deduction (less than two percent) from the employee's base pay plus an equal contribution from the hospital; there is an annual Christmas party and the Japanese annual tradition of gift giving. In many departments there are periodic parties where the staff, often under the influence of some sake, can air grievances and then return to work the next day as if nothing had happened. There are suggestion boxes around the hospital, but they yield less than 75 suggestions per year and most of these are not of great value. A weekly bulletin is distributed to 300 employees, and recently a 20-person "quality circle" was established, but it has not yielded any concrete suggestions. It should be noted that while suggestions are encouraged, no particular incentive (such as time off or a financial reward) is built into the suggestion system.

It is clear that personnel is a department central to the functioning of the hospital and one that is in touch with what is happening throughout the institution. Perhaps one can summarize the involvement of the personnel department at St. Luke's by noting that several times each week the personnel manager leaves his office and walks through the hospital to talk with staff and provide them with informal access to him.

DISCUSSION

One can argue, with some justification, that St. Luke's is unique among Japanese hospitals. Clearly it is an institution that actively pursues excellence in medical care. Perhaps the best illustration of this pursuit of excellence is the procedure in radiology of returning both the report and the X-ray to the initiating physician. The hospital is also unique in that its roots are in the American system of medical care and that by some standards, in particular, average length of stay, it is more successful than other Japanese hospitals. Of course, there are costs associated with shorter lengths of stay; at St. Luke's, staffing ratios are twice those of similar institutions. Another dimension of the hospital's uniqueness is that it has both its own nurse training program as well as a close relationship with a second program.

On the other hand, in some respects, St. Luke's is not so unique. All of its staff are Japanese, and the physicians, nurses, and technical staff all went through Japanese schools and were socialized to the values and norms of Japanese medical care and Japanese society. So, as noted earlier, St. Luke's offers a fascinating blend, and perhaps illustrates the tension, between East and West.

High-Quality Management

In terms of management, one must be particularly impressed with the quality and direction of the orientation program. The intensive involvement of so many levels of staff, as well as the respect shown the new employees, is unusual. Clearly, the message being given to the new staff is that they are now important and welcome members of the organization.

The employee evaluation system appears to provide management with the necessary information to sort out staff who are presenting problems as well as those who might be promoted sometime in the future. However, there is an issue related to providing feedback to the employee that deserves some attention. While some feedback is provided via the bonus, there is no direct mechanism for an employee to learn about his or her strengths and weaknesses. Whether a direct feedback system would be too threatening or damaging to relationships within the Japanese social system is a question deserving consideration.

Within the management team one does see a *ringi* system. For example, when the personnel manager wanted to initiate a new advertising campaign to recruit nurses, the request was sent around on a form, so that the various involved managerial staff could comment on the proposal before a final decision was made. The final signed form is documentation that the process was followed. In part, *ringi* is necessary at St. Luke's and other organizations where a central budgeting system is in place. In a decentralized system personnel would have an advertising budget, and the need for at least the budgetary approval portion of the *ringi* would be unnecessary.

Investment in Nursing Education

One is also struck by St. Luke's investment in nursing education—much of it to train nurses who will leave within several years. A limited cost-benefit analysis of hospital graduates indicates that, after considering the cost of alternate staff, the cost of the nursing programs, and the income generated by tuition and government subsidy, the hospital loses money by employing its own graduates. Would the hospital be better off recruiting nurses from outside schools? Or would it do well to more aggressively recruit students from Tokyo for its own schools? These are questions that also require consideration.

In the literature on Japanese management, much is made of the employees' commitment to suggesting change for the organization's betterment. Evidence of this level of employee interest was not present at St. Luke's or at any other hospital visited. The problem may be unrelated to employee interest but rather to the general boredom of seeing the same suggestion box every day. One option might be temporary suggestion boxes that are put in place during quarterly, focused campaigns. For example, one might have a cost containment or safety theme for the campaign and provide incentives for good suggestions such as theater tickets or monetary gifts. Quality circles are being considered, but plans are moving along slowly, and some management staff have voiced concern about their potential usefulness.

The lack of physician involvement in many activities was disappointing. Like their colleagues in the United States, Japanese physicians are placed on a financial and spiritual pedestal. They are too far removed from the "team" of hospital workers, even if they do belong to the same union. For example, at St. Luke's there is a four-day orientation for new staff, but the physicians and dentists have their own separate orientation. When do they become integrated members of the hospital work force? Despite being full-time, salaried staff, the answer may be never.

Toward the Future—Building a New Facility

A final point relates to the hospital's physical plant. St. Luke's is in a charming, warm, and tired building. Either extensive renovations and additions have to be made or a new replacement facility must be built. Based on numerous discussions, it appears that the latter course will be followed, with appropriate data collection and analysis now under way.

The long delays in starting the building project, plus the opening of the expanded neighboring hospital, may be taking a toll on the staff. What can be done about this is an open question. Perhaps, in a very un-Japanese way, some action is necessary. For example, the hospital could start construction of part of the new facility, such as the radiology, administration, or laboratory wing, and link it by tunnels or ramps to the present facility. This would, no doubt, involve obtaining zoning variances, but management must often engage in the art of the impossible. It is clear that some sense of movement about the new facility is necessary.

St. Luke's is a hospital with a wide constituency and an outstanding reputation. Its future will depend on the extent to which it can capitalize on its valuable assets and develop a new facility and system that can meet the challenges of the next several decades.

Chapter 8

Hospital Workers' Attitudes and Opinions in Japan and the United States

INTRODUCTION

A careful reading of the three case studies of the Japanese hospitals, presented in Chapters 5, 6, and 7, raises the possibility that there may indeed be an important difference in the attitudes and opinions of Japanese hospital workers and American hospital workers toward many facets of their work and worklife. This observation suggested the need to document these differences through the mechanism of a comparative survey, albeit an exploratory one.

This chapter reports the results of that survey, which was conducted in three Japanese and three American hospitals. The Japanese hospitals in the survey were the same hospitals described in the case studies. The three American hospitals are all located on the Eastern seaboard, but in different cities. One institution identified in this report as Cosmopolitan is a 300-bed voluntary hospital affiliated with a local medical school. It is located in an area similar to St. Luke's in that the daytime population of the primary service area is considerably greater than the evening and weekend population. The second American hospital (identified as Metropolitan) is a 600-bed voluntary hospital located in another metropolitan area; it is the primary teaching hospital of a well-known medical school. This hospital is similar to the Public Corporation Hospital in a variety of ways, including size and high-technology orientation. The third American hospital, Doctors', is a small proprietary hospital, similar in size and structure to the Kitashinagawa Hospital, the Japanese proprietary hospital. The primary service areas of the Japanese and American proprietary hospitals are strikingly similar in that they are both located at the fringes of a city, in a working class neighborhood.

METHODOLOGICAL NOTES AND LIMITATIONS

Before proceeding with a review of the findings, a number of methodological issues should be discussed. To begin, cross-cultural studies always present methodological problems on a variety of levels, including lingual and social constructs. These are serious and interrelated problems. In this research, an attempt was made to minimize these problems by using a number of questions conceptually similar to those that had been employed in other studies comparing attitudes of workers in Japanese firms with those of workers in American firms.

The questions, which were initially developed and modified at an American university, required translation into colloquial Japanese. This was accomplished by a bilingual senior health services researcher at Japan's National Institute of Hospital Administration. In a more elegant study design (and a more expensive one), the questionnaire would be retranslated into English to be certain that the questions had not lost their original meaning in the translation. Perhaps because this retranslation did not occur, there are some subtle differences in the Japanese and English versions of the questionnaire. For example, in the introduction to the questionnaire there is a statement that says the responses will be kept confidential. The Japanese word used to translate confidential is "secret." Is there a difference between confidential and "secret"?

Other methodological issues of considerable importance are sample size and quality of the sample. These variables affect the researcher's ability to generalize from results and confidence in the data-based findings. Theoretically, the sample should be an accurate reflection of the population under review. Failure to obtain an accurate sample necessarily limits the import that can be attached to the empirical data. As is indicated in the following paragraphs, many sampling problems were encountered, and these problems do represent an important limitation on the value of the data.

Obtaining Hospital Cooperation

Cooperation from the three American hospitals was easily obtained after a series of phone conversations and correspondence. The hospitals were selected because of their likely willingness to participate and the earlier-noted similarities between the general communities they serve and the communities served by the Japanese hospitals. There were no problems in eliciting responses from the three American hospitals; however, in two of the three hospitals the sample size was less than requested. The researcher, however, maintained no control over the sample selection other than to provide the senior administrative staff person with a sampling plan.

The Japanese hospitals were somewhat more problematic. In the first Japanese hospital surveyed, objections were raised to the questionnaire. Several members of top management felt that raising issues related to job satisfaction was likely to cause employees to become dissatisfied. One person made the analogy that "it is like asking a person to talk about the weaknesses of his father." Negotiations over the questionnaire often sounded like a debate at the United Nations where neither party cares to mention the subject or terms. Hours of discussion were held on extraneous topics, with my translator holding in check my attempts to discuss the questionnaire, saying it was not yet time. When the time did finally come, I was told that my sample size and distribution were acceptable but that the hospital's business manager would select the sample—not an elegant design, but a diplomatic solution. At this hospital (Public Corporation), the respondents were older and more likely to be in middle management positions than at the other hospitals.

In the second Japanese hospital, we encountered nurses who objected to some of the questions. Discussions and quiet diplomacy carried the day, and in this case, nurses who objected to a particular question were excused from answering it. No similar problems with specific questions, or the questionnaire in general, were encountered in the third hospital. However, it must be noted that in all three Japanese hospitals and all three American hospitals, the samples were essentially selected by someone in management. Despite this possible bias, the results do not indicate uniformity of opinion on most issues covered in the questionnaire. Thus, we feel somewhat confident that the respondents answered the questions in a forthright manner, without management's influence.

Obviously, the data are limited by the above-noted limitations, plus several technical problems. Thus, if the survey is approached as a definitive comparative analysis, it must be found wanting. However, if it is approached from the perspective of a pilot survey that provides clarifying and amplifying information about the case studies, its value is significantly enhanced,

The original plan for the data analysis called for sophisticated techniques such as factor analysis and regression analysis but was abandoned after the reality of the sample became evident. Because of the limitations inherent in the data, it was reasoned that the use of more sophisticated techniques would tend only to obscure the quality of the data. Therefore, what is presented in this chapter is essentially descriptive and comparative in nature. The data do point toward some tentative conclusions and hypotheses that should be useful in the development of future research projects. The survey questionnaire is reproduced as Exhibit 8-1.

Exhibit 8-1 Hospital Staff Survey

Instructions:

This survey is being administered to different groups of hospital employees in the United States and Japan as part of a research project being conducted by Professor Seth B. Goldsmith of the University of Massachusetts. Your responses to these questions will be treated in a confidential manner and no individual responses will be reported back to any hospital. Your cooperation in filling out this questionnaire is appreciated.

1. Age _____
2. Sex (circle one): male   female
3. Marital status (circle one): married   divorced   single   widowed
4. Number of children _____
5. *Education*
   a. Are you a high school graduate? (circle one)   yes   no
   b. Are you a nursing school graduate? (circle one)   yes   no
   c. Are you a college graduate? (circle one)   yes   no
   d. Did you go to a technical school to study a health profession? (circle one) yes   no
   e. Do you hold health-related licenses or registrations? (circle one)   yes   no
6. *Employment*
   a. What is your present job title? _____
   b. How many years have you been working at this hospital? _____
   c. How important were the following factors in your deciding to work at this hospital? (check one column for each factor)

Factors	Very Important	Important	Not Important
Pay scale			
Location of hospital			
Loyalty to the hospital because it trained me			
Friends who work here			
The reputation of the hospital			
The quality of medical care at the hospital			
Opportunity for professional advancement here			

Exhibit 8-1 continued

Factors	Very Important	Important	Not Important
Fringe benefits			
The timing of this job offer			
The need for my spouse to move to this area			

d. Under what circumstances would you consider leaving your present job at this hospital?

	Would definitely leave	Would look for another job	Do not know what I would do	Would definitely not leave
1. If the coworkers in your unit were not willing to socialize with you.				
2. If you were offered the same job with more money at a neighboring hospital.				
3. If you were offered the same job at the same money but closer to home.				
4. If your supervisor was fair to you but refused to socialize with you.				
5. If the medical staff treated you in an unpleasant way.				

Exhibit 8-1 continued

	Would definitely leave	Would look for another job	Do not know what I would do	Would definitely not leave
6. If important decisions were made about your work unit and your opinion was not solicited.				
7. If changes were occurring in your work unit and you were the last person in the unit to hear about them.				
8. If the hospital was running into serious financial problems and it seemed that you might lose your job within the next few months.				
9. If your hospital eliminated fringe benefits such as trips or clubs.				
10. If you felt that you had an unfair evaluation by your supervisor.				
11. If you were unfairly punished for something you did not do.				
12. If the hospital hired a person to work with you who was not qualified.				

Exhibit 8-1 continued

	Would definitely leave	Would look for another job	Do not know what I would do	Would definitely not leave
13. If after asking your supervisor for more responsibility you were not given it.				
14. If your shift was changed.				
15. If you felt the services provided to the patients were of poor quality.				
16. If you learned that the hospital you worked for was almost bankrupt.				

e. Please indicate whether you agree, disagree, or do not have an answer to the following questions.

	Agree	?	Disagree
At this hospital, management is doing its best to give us good working conditions.			
If I have a suggestion to make I feel free to talk to my supervisor about it.			
The administration tells staff about what is going on in the hospital.			
I have a great deal of interest in this hospital and its future.			

Exhibit 8-1 continued

	Agree	?	Disagree
I have confidence in the fairness and honesty of management.			
You can get fired at this hospital without just cause.			
I think this hospital's employee benefit program is OK.			
Hospital administration ignores complaints that come from employees.			

SAMPLE AGE DIFFERENCES

Table 8-1 displays the differences in age of the various samples, by hospital and work group. In one of the American hospitals, Doctors' Hospital, the statistic presented is only an estimate, because two of the five nurses gave their ages only as 40 + . In the other two American hospitals, the nurses' mean age differed by only three years. However, in the Japanese hospitals the age range is rather wide, with St. Luke's nurses the youngest and Public Corporation's nurses having a mean age almost twice that of the St. Luke's nurses. Also, at the Public Corporation Hospital the standard deviation is quite small, indicating that the dispersion around the mean age was quite narrow.

In the category of other staff, the mean age is similar among the three American hospitals and two of the Japanese hospitals. The third Japanese hospital, Public Corporation, has a dramatically higher mean age as well as a lower standard deviation.

The mean age data points up one of the problems with the sample, that is, to some degree, a lack of comparability. For example, nurses age 49, with perhaps 25 to 30 years' experience, might have a rather different view of the world than those who grew up a generation later. On the other hand, of the 12 sample

Table 8-1 Sample Age Differences Between U.S. and Japanese Hospitals

Hospital	Nurses (N =) Mean Age S.D.			Others (N =) Mean Age S.D.		
St. Luke's	(N = 30)	25.16	6.32	(N = 19)	30.52	8.07
Kitashinagawa	(N = 25)	31.95	9.30	(N = 20)	31.00	13.09
Public Corp.	(N = 14)	49.08	3.22	(N = 19)	49.26	5.45
Metropolitan	(N = 20)	35.16	10.18	(N = 24)	29.36	5.64
Doctors'	(N = 5)*	44.00	13.49	(N = 22)	33.42	12.51
Cosmopolitan	(N = 14)	32.46	7.77	(N = 21)	33.86	8.75

*Two of the five nurses at Doctors' Hospital listed their ages as 40+. For the purposes of these calculations, they were assumed to be 45 years old, producing a mean age of 44. If one assumed an average age for these two nurses of 50, then the mean would move up to 46 years.

groups—nurses and others at the 6 hospitals—9 of the groups, representing 83 percent of the sample, are clearly in the same generational category, with a mean age range of 25 to 35. This, too, can be a limiting factor since the population under study may not be representative of the total employee population at the hospitals. However, the size of the standard deviation in many of the sample groups suggests that the data may represent a somewhat broader cross section of the population than the mean age data might indicate.

SELECTING A PLACE TO WORK

One section of the questionnaire attempted to look at what factors were important to Japanese and American hospital workers in selecting a hospital where they would work. Theoretically, the Japanese worker's decision should be more important because of the likelihood of staying at one hospital over one's entire worklife; on the other hand, in the United States the expectation is for high turnover. In the survey, respondents were asked to answer a question regarding the importance of ten different factors in their decision to work at their present hospital. Possible responses were "very important," "important," and "not important." In this analysis, the categories of important and very important were combined, since both were clearly positive responses.

Attitudes of Japanese Workers

As Table 8-2 indicates, in all three Japanese hospitals reputation and quality of medical care are viewed as the most important factors in the decision. In two of the hospitals pay scale is a top-rated factor, and only at St. Luke's is loyalty because of training at the hospital rated high. The Public Corporation Hospital also has a nursing school, but the nursing staff did not consider this a significant factor even though the vast majority of the hospital's nurses are hired from its school. Clearly of least importance is the need to be in the area because of a spouse. This is a function of the small number of nurses in the sample who were married and that all the hospitals were located in a metropolitan area, where other jobs are generally available.

Timing also ranked low in two of the three hospitals; this is also a function of the Japanese system, where almost all new employees start at the same time each year. The American experience of job hunting and job hiring throughout the year is the exception, rather than the rule, in Japan.

The other staff who responded to the questionnaire, in Japan and the United States, tended to be a mix of technical employees (such as X-ray or laboratory technicians) and clerical or administrative staff. Table 8-3 provides a view of how these Japanese employees ranked the various factors. Quality of medical care was the first-ranked factor at two of the hospitals and third ranked at the other. At the Public Corporation Hospital, opportunity for professional advancement was the

---

Table 8-2 Nurses' Views of the Importance of Various Factors in Deciding Where to Work (Japan)

| Factor | *Percent Who Viewed Factor as Important* | | |
	St. Luke's	Kitashinagawa	Pub. Corp.
Quality of medical care at hospital	96%	92%	100%
Reputation of hospital	83	83	100
Fringe benefits	43	67	85
Pay scale	36	63	77
Timing of the offer	20	58	69
Location of hospital	50	58	54
Opportunity for professional advancement at hospital	36	41	63
Loyalty to hospital because it trained me	53	10	33
Friends who work at hospital	46	8	30
Need to be in area because of spouse	0	8	18

Table 8-3 Staff's (Other Than Nurses') Views of the Importance of Various Factors in Deciding Where to Work (Japan)

Factor	Percent Who Viewed Factor as Important		
	St. Luke's	Kitashinagawa	Pub. Corp.
Quality of medical care at hospital	84%	96%	64%
Reputation of hospital	84	96	55
Fringe benefits	26	80	50
Pay scale	63	85	73
Timing of the offer	68	68	14
Location of hospital	50	75	36
Opportunity for professional advancement at hospital	21	76	90
Loyalty to hospital because it trained me	5	5	0
Friends who work at hospital	10	28	20
Need to be in area because of spouse	10	22	17

highest ranked factor. This is partially because many of those responding to the survey were employees of the parent corporation, on rotation to the hospital but with no future at the hospital. Rather, their future was with the parent corporation and their present job was simply the right professional move in their climb up the corporate hierarchy. At the other hospitals, the employees most likely were making a career choice to work in hospitals. At St. Luke's, timing was the second-ranked factor, followed closely by pay scale. At the other hospitals timing was at the middle or bottom of the ranking, and pay scale was closer to the top.

Attitudes of American Workers

Now we can turn our attention to the nurses at the three American hospitals (Table 8-4). At the first hospital, Metropolitan, the nurses ranked quality of medical care first, along with fringe benefits; pay scale was a close second. Professional opportunity was ranked third and hospital reputation fourth. Reputation, so closely linked with quality in Japan, does not appear to be so linked at Metropolitan. At the bottom of the list are friends and spouse.

At the second hospital, Doctors', the sample is very small (N = 5), and it appears that the top ranking is shared by location, reputation, quality, and fringe benefits. Pay scale is in second place, and timing and spouse are at the bottom of the list.

Table 8-4 Nurses' Views of the Importance of Various Factors in
Deciding Where to Work (U.S.)

Factor	Percent Who Viewed Factor as Important		
	Metro.	Doctors'	Cosmo.
Quality of medical care at hospital	95%	100%	85%
Reputation of hospital	80	100	85
Fringe benefits	95	100	92
Pay scale	90	80	85
Timing of the offer	70	40	85
Location of hospital	75	100	85
Opportunity for professional advancement at hospital	85	60	85
Loyalty to hospital because it trained me	55	60	28
Friends who work at hospital	35	80	28
Need to be in area because of spouse	40	20	14

At the third American hospital, Cosmopolitan, the nurses ranked fringe benefits highest, with six other factors in second place: pay scale, location, reputation, quality, professional opportunity, and timing. Loyalty and needing to be in the area because of spouse were ranked at the bottom. Cosmopolitan, like St. Luke's, is located in a busy part of a large city, an area where housing and parking are both difficult to find. One of Cosmopolitan's important fringe benefits is the subsidized housing and free parking for nurses.

Table 8-5 summarizes the findings for staff other than nurses at the American hospitals. For the Metropolitan staff, pay scale was the number one reason for selecting the hospital as a place of work. Four factors ranked in second place: reputation, quality, professional opportunity, and the timing of the offer. Fringe benefits ranked third; 88 percent of the employees considered it important. Not until the fourth-ranked factor, hospital's location, is there a large drop in the percentage of persons who considered it important. The least important factors were loyalty because of training and friends.

At Doctors' Hospital, the staff other than nurses ranked fringe benefits as the top priority, followed closely by hospital location and timing of the job offer. Of least importance were loyalty because of training and needs of a spouse.

For the staff other than nurses at Cosmopolitan, fringe benefits were of highest importance, followed closely by pay scale, opportunity for professional advancement, and timing. Loyalty, friends, and spouse were at the bottom of the list of factors important in the selection decision.

Table 8-5 Staffs' (Other Than Nurses') Views of the Importance of Various Factors in Deciding Where to Work (U.S.)

	Percent Who Viewed Factor as Important		
Factor	*Metro.*	*Doctors'*	*Cosmo.*
Quality of medical care at hospital	92%	77%	80%
Reputation of hospital	92	77	65
Fringe benefits	88	90	95
Pay scale	96	81	90
Timing of the offer	92	86	85
Location of hospital	68	86	70
Opportunity for professional advancement at hospital	92	72	85
Loyalty to hospital because it trained me	32	50	45
Friends who work at hospital	32	22	40
Need to be in area because of spouse	52	9	5

CHI-SQUARE ANALYSIS

Since nurses were the most homogeneous of the work groups studied, a chi-square analysis was performed in order to compare the opinions of the Japanese and American nurses. Table 8-6 summarizes these findings and indicates there were five areas where significant differences were found: the importance of fringe benefits, pay scale, location, professional opportunities, and the need to relocate to be near one's spouse. Two of these, fringe benefits and professional opportunities, had the strongest statistical significance (Tables 8-7 and 8-10). One might ask why fringe benefits are so important to the American nurse. There is no easy answer, but it may be that fringe benefits represent income or income offsets that are not heavily taxed, and they are of more tangible value to an American than a Japanese. A second explanation is that fringe benefits are almost universal in Japan and they may have lost some of their appeal because of familiarity. Professional opportunities might be explained in the same way, adding that in Japan one is often placed on a professional "escalator," thus progress is slow but steady. The availability of professional opportunities suggests a more open and flexible system, which no doubt appeals to the traditional American way of doing business. Tables 8-8, 8-9, and 8-11 present the other significant chi-square results.

Table 8-6 Chi-Square Analyses of Factors Involved in Nurses' Decisions to Select a Place to Work

Factor	Chi-Square*	Significance Level
Quality of medical care	.32	N.S.
Reputation	.86	N.S.
Fringe benefits	16.26	<.001
Pay scale	5.65	<.02
Timing of offer	.00093	N.S.
Location	2.9	<.10
Opportunity	14.59	<.001
Loyalty	2.139	N.S.
Friends	.3478	N.S.
Spouse	3.088	<.05

*All chi-squares are with 1 degree of freedom.

Table 8-7 The Importance of Fringe Benefits in Nurses' Decisions to Select a Place to Work

	Important	Not Important
United States	36	2
Japan	33	25

$X = 16.262$, 1 d.f., $p < .001$

Table 8-8 The Importance of Pay Scale in Nurses' Decisions to Select a Place to Work

	Important	Not Important
United States	34	5
Japan	45	23

$X = 5.65$, 1 d.f., $p < .02$

Table 8-9 The Importance of Location in Nurses' Decisions to Select a Place to Work

	Important	Not Important
United States	30	9
Japan	40	26

X = 2.9, 1 d.f., p < .10

Table 8-10 The Importance of Professional Opportunities in Nurses' Decisions to Select a Place to Work

	Important	Not Important
United States	37	7
Japan	25	33

X = 14.598, 1 d.f., p < .001

Table 8-11 The Importance of Needs of Spouse in Nurses' Decisions to Select a Place to Work

	Important	Not Important
United States	11	26
Japan	7	47

X = 3.88, 1 d.f., p < .05

In summary, despite the limitations identified earlier, the data suggest that among the Japanese nursing staffs there are some commonly shared opinions about what is important and unimportant in selecting a work place; among the American nurses, the commonly shared opinions cover a greater range of factors. The data also indicate the importance of a hospital's reputation and the quality of care that the hospital appears to offer.

JOB LEAVING ATTITUDES

In the next series of questions, staff at the three American hospitals and three Japanese hospitals were given a set of hypothetical questions and situations and asked if they would leave their present jobs if these situations occurred. The questionnaire allowed for these responses: would definitely leave, would look for another job, do not know what I would do, and would definitely not leave. In this analysis, the responses to "would definitely leave" and "would look for another job" were combined because of their obvious overlapping sentiment. A total of 16 questions were asked, but one question (number 12) was not included in the analysis because many respondents thought it confusing. The questions can be grouped into the following categories: coworker relations, hospital economic conditions, supervisory relationships, managerial climate, and hospital status.

Coworker Relationships

In the first category, coworker relationships, only one question was asked: What would you do "if the coworkers in your unit were not willing to socialize with you"?

The results are presented in Tables 8-12 and 8-13. Among the American hospital nurses, most would stay, although some were uncertain about what they would do. Among the nurses in the Japanese hospitals, there is a substantial difference in the responses. At Kitashinagawa, the majority would stay, and slightly more than a third were uncertain. At the Public Corporation Hospital,

---

Table 8-12 Effect of Poor Coworker Relationships on Job Leaving
Attitudes (Nurses)

	Would Leave	Uncertain	Wouldn't Leave
St. Luke's	10%	73%	16%
Kitashinagawa	4	36	60
Public Corp.	7	54	39
Metropolitan	15	30	55
Doctors'	20	40	40
Cosmopolitan	7	29	64

Table 8-13 Effect of Poor Coworker Relationships on Job Leaving
Attitudes (Nonnursing Staff)

	Would Leave	*Uncertain*	*Wouldn't Leave*
St. Luke's	21%	26%	53%
Kitashinagawa	10	55	35
Public Corp.	25	75	0
Metropolitan	13	17	71
Doctors'	5	14	81
Cosmopolitan	5	14	81

slightly more than half were uncertain, and 38 percent would stay. But at St. Luke's, almost three-quarters of the staff were uncertain. The explanation may have to do with the closeness of the work groups at St. Luke's and the relationships that have been nurtured through shared nursing school and dormitory living experiences. Such relationships, if broken, may be too painful to endure, thus resulting in the nurses' uncertainty.

The data for the staff other than nurses (Table 8-13) indicates that for the American workers, lack of socialization would not be a problem. On the other hand, in the Japanese hospitals (particularly Kitashinagawa and Public Corporation) problems with coworker relationships might cause turnover and create a state of uncertainty.

Managerial Climate

The second category examined under job leaving attitudes is described as managerial climate (Tables 8-14, 8-15, 8-16, and 8-17). In this category, staff were asked what they would do in the following five circumstances: (1) if the medical staff treated them in an unpleasant way; (2) if important decisions were made about their work unit and their opinion was not solicited; (3) if changes occurred in their work unit and they were the last to hear about them; (4) if they were unfairly punished for something they did not do; and (5) if their shift was changed. At all three Japanese hospitals, the data suggest that unfair punishment is the only managerial climate element that would cause the nurses to seriously look for another job, although a majority of nurses would be in some state of looking or uncertainty if the other problems manifested themselves.

Table 8-14 Managerial Climate and Job Leaving Attitudes of Nurses at Japanese Hospitals

Factor	Would Leave			Uncertain			Wouldn't Leave		
	SL	KS	PC	SL	KS	PC	SL	KS	PC
Medical staff treats you unpleasantly	6%	0%	7%	33%	20%	46%	56%	80%	46%
Opinion not solicited about important work unit changes	20	8	15	56	28	62	21	64	23
Changes made in work unit and you find out last	17	8	0	40	20	69	40	72	31
Unfair punishment for something not done	50	36	31	33	32	54	17	32	15
If shift is changed	17	4	0	50	12	46	33	84	54

Note: SL = St. Luke's
      KS = Kitashinagawa
      PC = Public Corporation

Table 8-15 Managerial Climate and Job Leaving Attitudes of Nurses at American Hospitals

Factor	Would Leave			Uncertain			Wouldn't Leave		
	MP	DO	CS	MP	DO	CS	MP	DO	CS
Medical staff treats you unpleasantly	20%	0%	36%	20%	60%	21%	60%	40%	43%
Opinion not solicited about important work unit changes	35	20	64	35	40	21	30	40	14
Changes made in work unit and you find out last	15	20	50	45	20	21	40	60	29
Unfair punishment for something not done	60	40	64	20	20	14	15	40	21
If shift is changed	55	60	85	20	20	7	25	20	7

Note: MP = Metropolitan
      DO = Doctors'
      CS = Cosmopolitan

Table 8-16 Managerial Climate and Job Leaving Attitudes of Staff Other Than Nurses at Japanese Hospitals

Factor	Would Leave			Uncertain			Wouldn't Leave		
	SL	KS	PC	SL	KS	PC	SL	KS	PC
Medical staff treats you unpleasantly	11%	10%	0%	32%	25%	23%	58%	60%	77%
Opinion not solicited about important work unit changes	11	0	23	53	55	0	37	45	77
Changes made in work unit and you find out last	11	5	23	27	30	8	63	65	69
Unfair punishment for something not done	37	45	31	37	25	23	26	30	46
If shift is changed	0	15	0	63	35	23	37	45	77

Table 8-17 Managerial Climate and Job Leaving Attitudes of Staff Other Than Nurses at American Hospitals

Factor	Would Leave			Uncertain			Wouldn't Leave		
	MP	DO	CS	MP	DO	CS	MP	DO	CS
Medical staff treats you unpleasantly	29%	5%	19%	29%	41%	33%	42%	55%	48%
Opinion not solicited about important work unit changes	17	14	29	42	23	38	42	64	29
Changes made in work unit and you find out last	21	18	33	38	32	19	42	50	48
Unfair punishment for something not done	42	9	29	29	72	43	33	18	29
If shift is changed	21	0	38	29	45	24	29	55	24

At both the Public Corporation and Kitashinagawa Hospitals the problem of unfair punishment has the strongest potential for causing a person to leave the job. At Kitashinagawa, however, the nurses showed a relatively greater reluctance to leave than at the other two hospitals. A possible explanation is that the workers have a greater sense of personal involvement at Kitashinagawa because the hospital is broken up into small independent facilities. The other two hospitals are relatively large and, perhaps, somewhat less personal.

The attitudes of the American nurses (Table 8-15) are in sharp contrast to the attitudes of their Japanese counterparts. In general, the data from the two voluntary hospitals, Cosmopolitan and Metropolitan, demonstrate that the components of managerial climate are quite important to the nurses. For example, at Cosmopolitan 35 percent of the staff indicated that they would leave if treated unpleasantly by the medical staff, and 85 percent of the nurses questioned at that hospital said they would leave if their shift were changed. Even at Doctors', with the smallest sample, a majority of nurses said they would leave if there was a shift change. The pattern seen in response to the unfair punishment question is similar among both the Japanese and American nurses. An interesting question is, why do the American nurses feel so much more strongly about these managerial climate issues than their Japanese counterparts? A possible explanation might be that American nurses have greater job mobility and are thus more reluctant to stay in a position filled with the problems and irritants identified as managerial climate. A second explanation that might be related to the strong feelings about shift changes is that the American nurse may have primary commitments outside of the job (to a family unit) and work must be of secondary importance. In such a situation, shift changes may be viewed as too disruptive to family life and a reasonable justification for resignation. Finally, one might posit that the American nurses take only the short run view because of the tenuous nature of their jobs. The Japanese nurse, with her lifetime employment and long-term commitment to the organization, can afford to put up with somewhat more inequitable treatment, and perhaps abuse, because she knows that she can eventually prevail if she waits her turn and she remains a supporter of the group. The American's more individualistic style does not allow for such patience.

The data from the staff other than nurses show the same general pattern described earlier but not with the same strength. It is clear that an adverse managerial climate would cause a higher percentage of American than Japanese workers to leave or to experience a state of uncertainty. Once again, unfair punishment is the most important reason people think about leaving their jobs.

Supervisory Relationships

The next category examined under job leaving attitudes focused on supervisory relationships. The three questions in this category asked respondents what they would do (1) if their supervisor was fair to them but refused to socialize with them; (2) if they felt they had received an unfair evaluation by their supervisor; and (3) if, after asking their supervisor for more responsibility, they were not given it. The data indicate that for the nurses at the Japanese hospitals (Table 8-18), an unfair evaluation is the strongest impetus to leave or to move into a state of uncertainty. In the American hospitals (Table 8-20), the same pattern is repeated. The answers presented by the other workers at all three Japanese hospitals (Table 8-19) demonstrate the relative weakness of supervisory problems as a reason for leaving, although an unfair evaluation—or a supervisor unwilling to give an employee more responsibility—will generate a high degree of uncertainty. For the American

Table 8-18 Supervisory Relationships and Job Leaving Attitudes of Nurses at Japanese Hospitals

Factor	Would Leave			Uncertain			Would Not Leave		
	SL	KS	PC	SL	KS	PC	SL	KS	PC
Fair supervisor who refused to socialize	0%	4%	8%	40%	28%	38%	60%	68%	54%
Unfair evaluation by supervisor	30	16	0	56	36	62	13	48	23
Supervisor unwilling to give more responsibility	10	4	8	46	28	46	43	68	46

Table 8-19 Supervisory Relationships and Job Leaving Attitudes of Staff Other Than Nurses at Japanese Hospitals

Factor	Would Leave			Uncertain			Would Not Leave		
	SL	KS	PC	SL	KS	PC	SL	KS	PC
Fair supervisor who refused to socialize	0%	5%	0%	26%	45%	31%	74%	50%	69%
Unfair evaluation by supervisor	21	15	15	42	65	8	32	20	0
Supervisor unwilling to give more responsibility	11	5	15	37	50	38	53	45	46

Table 8-20 Supervisory Relationships and Job Leaving Attitudes of Nurses at American Hospitals

Factor	Would Leave			Uncertain			Would Not Leave		
	MP	DO	CS	MP	DO	CS	MP	DO	CS
Fair supervisor who refused to socialize	5%	40%	0%	5%	0%	7%	90%	60%	93%
Unfair evaluation by supervisor	30	40	29	40	20	29	30	40	36
Supervisor unwilling to give more responsibility	25	40	29	30	40	29	45	20	43

nonnursing workers (Table 8-21), we see a pattern similar to that of the Japanese hospital workers.

The data also suggest that the American nurse is more likely to be disturbed over the issue of additional responsibility than her Japanese counterpart; we need to consider why this is such an important issue. Perhaps it is related to the notion that the Japanese nurse, with her permanent employment status and escalating salary, is not worried about a temporary setback because she has a longer term view and commitment than her American counterpart.

Table 8-21 Supervisory Relationships and Job Leaving Attitudes of Staff Other Than Nurses at American Hospitals

Factor	Would Leave			Uncertain			Would Not Leave		
	MP	DO	CS	MP	DO	CS	MP	DO	CS
Fair supervisor who refused to socialize	0%	0%	0%	8%	5%	14%	92%	9%	48%
Unfair evaluation by supervisor	17	5	29	29	41	24	54	55	48
Supervisor unwilling to give more responsibility	25	5	24	33	32	33	46	64	43

Economic Conditions

The fourth category examined under job leaving attitudes was that of economic conditions. Staff were asked what they would do under the following five circumstances: (1) if they were offered the same job, with more money, at a neighboring hospital; (2) if they were offered the same job, at the same salary, but closer to home; (3) if the hospital were running into serious financial problems and it seemed they might lose their job within the next few months; (4) if the hospital eliminated fringe benefits such as trips or clubs; and (5) if they learned that the hospital they worked for was almost bankrupt.

The data from the Japanese nurses (Table 8-22) indicate that if the hospital's economic situation was poor, they would seriously think of leaving. While the prospect of lost fringe benefits was relatively unimportant, the possibility of a higher paying job or lower costs (through a job closer to home) would cause many Japanese nurses to contemplate leaving. Comparing nurses to other workers at the same hospitals (Table 8-23), we see a fairly similar picture, except at the Public Corporation Hospital. However, it should be noted that many of the respondents in the other category at that hospital perceive themselves more as employees of the corporation than the hospital, and the loyalty to that profitable and successful parent enterprise likely transcends loyalty to the hospital.

The picture at the American hospitals (Table 8-24) is that of nurses who are loyal, but not to the point of probable economic deprivation. At two of the three

---

Table 8-22 Economic Conditions and Job Leaving Attitudes of Nurses at Japanese Hospitals

Factor	Would Leave			Uncertain			Would Not Leave		
	SL	KS	PC	SL	KS	PC	SL	KS	PC
Same job, more money, neighboring hospital	3%	8%	0%	70%	36%	85%	26%	56%	15%
Same job, same money, closer to home	7	20	15	53	28	69	36	52	0
Hospital in economic trouble, might lose job in few months	70	36	46	23	40	46	6	20	8
Hospital eliminates fringe benefits, trips, and clubs	3	4	0	43	20	38	53	76	62
Hospital almost bankrupt	60	32	38	27	40	38	10	28	15

Table 8-23 Economic Conditions and Job Leaving Attitudes of Staff Other Than Nurses at Japanese Hospitals

Factor	Would Leave			Uncertain			Would Not Leave		
	SL	KS	PC	SL	KS	PC	SL	KS	PC
Same job, more money, neighboring hospital	16%	10%	0%	53%	50%	23%	32%	40%	77%
Same job, same money, closer to home	11	5	0	47	60	15	42	35	85
Hospital in economic trouble, might lose job in few months	68	50	31	16	35	38	16	15	31
Hospital eliminates fringe benefits, trips, and clubs	0	60	8	21	45	15	79	45	77
Hospital almost bankrupt	63	35	23	11	35	31	26	35	46

Table 8-24 Economic Conditions and Job Leaving Attitudes of Nurses at American Hospitals

Factor	Would Leave			Uncertain			Would Not Leave		
	MP	DO	CS	MP	DO	CS	MP	DO	CS
Same job, more money, neighboring hospital	40%	20%	43%	30%	40%	36%	30%	40%	21%
Same job, same money, closer to home	25	0	7	25	20	43	50	80	50
Hospital in economic trouble, might lose job in few months	85	60	71	10	0	14	5	40	14
Hospital eliminates fringe benefits, trips, and clubs	5	0	0	10	0	14	85	100	85
Hospital almost bankrupt	85	40	71	10	40	14	5	20	14

hospitals (Metropolitan and Cosmopolitan), a higher salary at a neighboring hospital would be an attractive offer; at Doctors' and Cosmopolitan, the distance factor wasn't very strong. Fringe benefits seem, for the most part, to be irrelevant. The nonnursing workers at the American hospitals (Table 8-25) present a picture

Table 8-25 Economic Conditions and Job Leaving Attitudes of Staff Other Than Nurses at American Hospitals

Factor	Would Leave			Uncertain			Would Not Leave		
	MP	DO	CS	MP	DO	CS	MP	DO	CS
Same job, more money, neighboring hospital	42%	23%	57%	46%	50%	29%	13%	27%	14%
Same job, same money, closer to home	38	5	33	25	18	24	33	77	43
Hospital in economic trouble, might lose job in few months	88	27	57	4	41	38	8	32	5
Hospital eliminates fringe benefits, trips, and clubs	4	0	14	0	5	5	96	50	71
Hospital almost bankrupt	83	32	57	17	27	29	0	41	10

that is quite similar at two of the three hospitals and rather different at Doctors', which is a small private hospital. Once again, the possible importance of increased personal involvement within a small organization may be a factor.

Inspection of the data reveals that the differences are primarily ones of degree. Fringe benefit loss, according to the American respondents, is rather unimportant, and in Japan it would only create a sense of uncertainty in most workers. Similarly, with regard to impending bankruptcy, the American nurse would bail out with alacrity, while a fair percentage of the Japanese would not leave but would be moved to a state of uncertainty.

Hospital Quality

The last item examined under job leaving attitudes was related to hospital quality. The question asked was, What would you do "if you felt the services provided to the patients were of poor quality"?

The data in Table 8-26 indicate that among nurses in the three American hospitals, problems in perceived quality would cause a fair percentage of staff to leave. For staff other than nurses (Table 8-27) the quality issue seemed slightly less important, perhaps reflecting their lack of involvement in direct patient care.

The data also clearly demonstrate that problems with quality would cause the St. Luke's nurses, but not those at Kitashinagawa, to leave. At the Public Corporation

Table 8-26 Effect of Poor Quality Medical Care on Job Leaving Attitudes (Nurses)

	Would Leave	Uncertain	Would Not Leave
St Luke's	63%	23%	13%
Kitashinagawa	20	32	48
Public Corp.	15	62	23
Metropolitan	65	20	15
Doctors'	20	40	40
Cosmopolitan	57	21	21

Table 8-27 Effect of Poor Quality Medical Care on Job Leaving Attitudes of Staff Other Than Nurses

	Would Leave	Uncertain	Would Not Leave
St Luke's	16%	53%	32%
Kitashinagawa	10	55	35
Public Corp.	8	8	84
Metropolitan	43	19	22
Doctors'	27	27	45
Cosmopolitan	35	25	40

Hospital, quality-related problems would result in the majority of nurses moving into a state of uncertainty. A possible explanation for the findings at St. Luke's may have to do with St. Luke's well-known commitment to excellence: the nurses come with high expectations, and disappointment might result in job leaving attitudes. In contrast, Kitashinagawa is not a teaching hospital, and perhaps the nurses there have a different perception of quality. Once again, and probably for the same reasons, the issue of quality does not appear to be as important to the nonnursing workers.

The next set of questions focused on the general attitudes of the employees toward the hospital and its administration. Respondents were asked to respond to a series of statements by indicating whether they agreed, disagreed, or had no answer. Of the eight questions in this section, five were directly related to the hospital's administration: (1) at this hospital, management is doing its best to give us good working conditions; (2) the administration tells the staff what is going on in the hospital; (3) I have confidence in the fairness and honesty of management; (4) you can get fired at this hospital without just cause; and (5) hospital administration ignores complaints that come from employees. One question focused on supervision: If I have a suggestion to make, I feel free to talk to my supervisor about it. And, finally, two questions considered the staff member's general view of the organization: (1) I have a great deal of interest in this hospital and its future; and (2) I think the hospital's employee benefit program is OK.

ATTITUDES TOWARD HOSPITAL ADMINISTRATION

Table 8-28 provides a summary of how the nurses at the three Japanese hospitals and three American hospitals viewed their hospital's administration. The data from Doctors' Hospital come from such a small sample ($N = 5$) that they should be discounted. Also, it should be noted that most of the nurses in the Public Corporation sample were in managerial positions.

In the American hospitals, the data suggest that the picture is mixed. For example, at Cosmopolitan and Metropolitan, between one-third and one-half of the nurses thought management was trying to provide good working conditions, be fair, and communicate with staff. None of the nurses believed that they might be

Table 8-28 Nurses' Opinions of Hospital Administration

	Percentage of Staff Who Agreed with the Following Statements					
	SL	KS	PC	MP	DO	CS
Hospital management is doing its best to give us good working conditions.	13%	76%	57%	50%	100%	43%
The administration tells staff what is going on.	26	72	57	45	80	36
I have confidence in the fairness and honesty of management.	13	60	50	30	60	57
You can get fired at this hospital without just cause.	6	15	0	15	0	0
Hospital administration ignores complaints.	3	16	7	35	0	7

Note: SL = St. Luke's   MP = Metropolitan
        KS = Kitashinagawa   DO = Doctors'
        PC = Public Corp.   CS = Cosmopolitan

fired arbitrarily, but at Metropolitan Hospital, a third said that management did ignore complaints. Table 8-29 examines the opinions of staff other than nurses, and in the American hospitals we see generally similar findings. However, for these employees the perception was that complaints were not ignored at Metropolitan, but were ignored at Cosmopolitan.

In two of the three Japanese hospitals, the data present a strongly favorable picture in terms of managerial concerns about working conditions, communications, and fairness and honesty. The just-cause-in-firing issue and ignoring complaints follow a pattern similar to that at the American hospitals, and the staff other than nurses voted similarly to the nurses. It should be noted that St. Luke's consistently appears to be the most poorly rated of the three hospitals. Possible explanations for this involve the poor physical state of the hospital, the perceived social distance of management, higher staff expectations, the relative age of the staff, and perhaps poor management practices.

ATTITUDES TOWARD SUPERVISION

Only one question was asked in the area of supervisory relationships, and the responses represent a mixed bag, with 85 percent of the Cosmopolitan nurses and 35 percent of the Metropolitan nurses agreeing that they felt free to make suggestions to their supervisors (Table 8-30). In the Japanese hospitals, 76 percent

---

Table 8-29 Staff's (Other Than Nurses') Opinions of Hospital Administration

	Percentage of Staff Who Agreed with the Following Statements					
	SL	KS	PC	MP	DO	CS
Hospital management is doing its best to give us good working conditions.	11%	50%	61%	44%	82%	33%
The administration tells staff what is going on.	32	45	55	56	56	29
I have confidence in the fairness and honesty of management.	32	40	72	32	5	33
You can get fired at this hospital without just cause.	5	5	0	12	36	10
Hospital administration ignores complaints.	11	5	0	12	9	33

Table 8-30 Nurses' Opinions About Supervisory Relationships

	Percentage of Staff Who Agreed with the Following Statement:					
	SL	*KS*	*PC*	*MP*	*DO*	*CS*
I feel free to make suggestions.	46%	76%	64%	35%	100%	85%

of the Kitashinagawa nurses but only 46 percent of the St. Luke's nurses agreed with the statement. When the same question was asked of the nonnursing workers (Table 8-31), we see a dramatic difference between the American hospitals, where between 88 percent and 95 percent of the staff agreed with the statement and two of the Japanese hospitals, St. Luke's and Kitashinagawa, where only 53 percent and 40 percent, respectively, agreed with the statement. At St. Luke's and the Public Corporation Hospital, the staff agreed with the statement to a greater degree than the nurses, but at Kitashinagawa, there is a large drop: 76 percent of the nurses there felt free to make suggestions but only 40 percent of the other staff.

OPINIONS ABOUT THE ORGANIZATION

The questions in this category looked at the employees' interest in the future of the organization and their perception of the fringe benefit program (Tables 8-32 and 8-33). In the American hospitals, a strong majority of the nurses and other staff expressed interest in the future of the hospital as did their counterparts in Japan, with the exception of the nurses at St. Luke's. Among this group, only 43 percent of the nurses agreed with the statement. Regarding the fringe benefit

Table 8-31 Staff's (Other Than Nurses') Opinions About Supervisory Relationships

	Percentage of Staff Who Agreed with the Following Statement					
	SL	*KS*	*PC*	*MP*	*DO*	*CS*
I feel free to make suggestions.	53%	40%	88%	88%	95%	95%

Table 8-32 Nurses' Opinions About the Organization

	Percentage of Staff Who Agreed with the Following Statements					
	SL	KS	PC	MP	DO	CS
I have a great deal of interest in this hospital and its future.	43%	84%	57%	70%	100%	93%
I think this hospital's employee benefit program is OK.	3	56	42	50	80	79

Table 8-33 Staff's (Other Than Nurses') Opinions About the Organization

	Percentage of Staff Who Agreed with the Following Statements					
	SL	KS	PC	MP	DO	CS
I have a great deal of interest in this hospital and its future.	84%	60%	94%	76%	68%	76%
I think this hospital's employee benefit program is OK.	5	30	50	80	41	62

programs, the American workers are apparently somewhat more satisfied than the Japanese workers. This is somewhat unexpected, considering the range of fringe benefits offered in Japan.

SUMMARY

This chapter began by looking at what factors were important to a sample of American and Japanese hospital workers in selecting a place to work. It continued by examining how relationships with coworkers, the managerial climate, supervisory relationships, economic conditions, and lastly, the quality of the hospitals' services might affect job leaving attitudes. Finally, the workers' opinions about hospital administration and their own interest in the institution were analyzed.

Despite the limitations of the data due to sampling problems, questionnaire design, and the inherent bias of an American seeking to answer questions about American hospital management by looking abroad, the results of the survey do suggest the importance of a hospital's reputation and quality in the initial selection of a workplace among Japanese hospital workers. While quality and reputation are also important in the United States, pay is cited more consistently as an important factor in the United States than in Japan.

In the area of job leaving attitudes, poor relationships with coworkers would appear to be more problematic for the Japanese than for Americans, while poor relationships with medical staff would prove a greater problem for Americans than for Japanese. Problems with management would also present more of a reason for the Americans, rather than the Japanese, to leave. Deteriorating economic conditions in the Japanese or American hospitals would be an incentive for most staff to start looking for new jobs. Finally, with regard to quality, Japanese and American nurses would seriously consider leaving if the quality of medical care started to decline in their hospitals.

The last area studied examined opinions toward the management of the hospitals. In general, most staff thought favorably of management, with one notable exception, and favorably of supervisory personnel. Workers showed a good deal of interest in the future of their organizations.

Together, the data from this survey paint an interesting, comparative picture of workers' attitudes and opinions in six hospitals. Perhaps what is most important is that there are differences among workers and hospitals, and for the astute manager, there are many ways to improve the quality of worklife of all hospital staff.

Co_

This final section of two chapters is in part a summary of the earlier eight chapters and an analysis of what we can learn from the Japanese experience.

The summary attempts to synthesize and discuss the material presented in the background chapters, the case studies, and the survey. It is really left for the final chapter to present a set of ideas that, if thoughtfully implemented, could have a profound impact on hospitals in this country. While these ideas represent significant departures from the way many hospital administrators presently manage their institutions, they also represent significant challenges for the future.

Part III

...clusions

Chapter 9

Summary and Discussion: Japanese Hospitals and Management

Although the fundamental interest in this volume is management, it is imperative to understand the context within which management operates in order to understand management itself. Toward these goals, this chapter presents conclusions on both management practices and the organization and delivery of health care services in Japanese hospitals.

THE JAPANESE HOSPITAL

Long-Term Care Role

The role of the general hospital is different in Japan than in the United States. In the United States, the general medical and surgical hospital is a short stay institution, where more than 50 percent of the patients stay less than 30 days. But in Japan, the concept of the acute care institution as it is defined in the United States does not exist. The average length of stay in Japanese hospitals is in excess of 30 days, and the Japanese hospital takes a greater responsibility for intermediate and long-term care than does its American counterpart. The extended care role results from the small number of nursing home beds in Japan (approximately 70,000); the cramped living quarters in Japanese homes (which makes it difficult for the recuperating patient to be treated under a home care program); and, as in all industrialized countries, the diminishing access to an extended family that could provide nursing-type care.

119

Medical Staff Organization

A second important difference between the Japanese hospital and its American counterpart is related to the organization of the medical staff. Almost without exception, Japanese hospitals operate with full-time medical staffs. The American approach, where attending staff physicians see patients in their private offices and admit the patients into a local hospital if necessary, does not exist in Japan. In Japan, the physician has basically three options: ambulatory care practice with no access to inpatient beds; ambulatory care practice with access to clinic beds (a clinic may have no more than 19 beds and patient stays are limited to 48 hours); or a hospital-based practice, where ambulatory care is delivered in an outpatient clinic and the physician has access to the hospital's beds.

Hospitals in Japan therefore all employ full-time medical staffs. Further, since they are competing with one another and the ambulatory care practitioners for patients, they must maintain large outpatient clinics in order to ensure a steady flow of inpatients. Under the present system in Japan, there is little incentive for an ambulatory care physician to refer a patient to a hospital; indeed, there are disincentives, such as the possibility that the physician will lose the patient entirely and will not be able to treat or bill the patient while hospitalized.

Staffing the Outpatient Clinic

The outpatient clinic is staffed by both the full-time medical staff and, in many hospitals, part-time, moonlighting physicians (often, the moonlighting physicians are medical school faculty). Theoretically, the physician staffing level in hospitals is one physician per 50 patients, with 3 outpatients counting as 1 inpatient. Regardless of staffing levels, there are long waits in outpatient departments, giving credence to a popular expression: "wait three hours and be seen for three minutes." The specifics of this problem were described to me by an American business consultant, fluent in Japanese, who visited a medical center outpatient clinic. On the initial visit, he waited three hours and saw the doctor for nine minutes. On the follow-up visit, there was a two-hour wait and a three-minute session with the doctor. On both visits he decided not to pick up his medications because of the extra hour wait at the hospital pharmacy. In discussing this problem with several Japanese colleagues, I was offered the following explanation. The Japanese patient would prefer to wait hours with the assurance of being seen—if the problem is not serious—than come back in two days for an appointment and a significantly shorter wait. Other views about these long waits include that (1) they are the hospitals' way of rationing the outpatient services (patients have to really want to be treated in the hospital, otherwise they would go to an ambulatory care doctor, where the waits are much shorter), and (2) they are caused by patients who shop around at different hospitals, looking for the best doctor for their condition.

Clearly, the organizational role of the physician and the functioning of medical staff within the hospital organization is different in Japan than in the United States or England. Unlike England, where the primary care practitioner functions as the gatekeeper to the hospital system or the United States, where the primary care practitioner has a close relationship with the community hospital, in Japan, the doctor is either part of the hospital (essentially, a full-time staff member) or completely outside the hospital system.

A striking organizational difference between American and Japanese hospitals is related to hospital ownership. While the private, for-profit hospitals are certainly making inroads in the United States, the level of private ownership is much less than in Japan. Perhaps of particular interest to Americans is the tradition of Japanese public hospitals that are renowned for their excellence.

National Health Insurance

Finally, it is necessary to recognize the significance of the national health insurance system in Japan and the effects of its attendant reimbursement scheme on hospital organization and management. Basically, hospitals are reimbursed on a per service basis, not directly related to the service's cost. Each service is worth a predetermined point value and each year, after extensive negotiations between the government and the providers, a yen value is placed on a point. The critical issue is that the point value for a service does not vary among hospitals; thus, in Japan, there are not the wide reimbursement disparities there are in the United States.

For patients, this means they effectively have a credit card with a set worth, regardless of the institution they are dealing with. On the other hand, additional payments for private rooms or other amenities provide some type of informal patient distribution system. The reimbursement system certainly rewards providers who can keep costs down (or run up costs where profit margins are high). Maintaining minimum staffing levels, prescribing and dispensing many drugs, ordering lab tests, and skimping on plant maintenance and capital improvements are sure ways of keeping a hospital in the black.

So, the hospital administrator in Japan has to cope with the following situation: The physical facility is like its American counterpart in appearances and is built to function as an acute care institution; however, relative to American hospitals, the Japanese facility will have a disproportionately large outpatient service. Patients receiving care there will be inpatients for three to four times as long as they would in the United States, but their care will cover a broad spectrum, from the acute to the recuperative phases. The administrator will have to manage a staff that includes a significant percentage of physicians, but the single largest professional group will be nurses. And finally, as noted earlier, reimbursement will encourage the staff, and hospital, to behave in certain revenue-maximizing and cost-minimizing fashions.

MANAGEMENT OF THE JAPANESE HOSPITAL

The Hospital Administrator

Who is responsible for management in the Japanese hospital? The Medical Services Act of Japan requires that all hospital administrators be physicians. The law is obeyed, and the post of hospital administrator is frequently combined with a clinical practice. Generally, the post is awarded to a very senior member of the medical staff (or the physician owner, in the case of private hospitals) whose involvement in decision making has probably been limited over the years. But this approach is in keeping with the general system of management in Japan, which stresses the value of the generalist and on-the-job training. In both corporation and hospital the practice prevails, and seniority is of paramount importance. In the university hospital, a distinguished senior professor becomes the hospital administrator; in the government hospital, it is a senior practitioner or retired professor. As noted before, the private hospital is most likely to have its owner as hospital administrator.

The Business Manager

Frequently, there is a business manager who assists the administrator. The role of the business manager is analogous to the assistant administrator for nonprofessional affairs in an American institution. Training for this position is usually accomplished through on-the-job learning, with an occasional short course. The proliferation of graduate health service and hospital administration courses that we see in the United States simply does not exist in Japan. By the same token, there are very few graduate degree programs in business in Japan. Thus, whether someone wants to become successful in a Japanese corporation or hospital, the route is the same: enter the organization after college (in some cases, after high school) and slowly work up the corporate ladder. Perhaps what is most interesting is that these nonphysician business managers have a rather restricted role, although some suggest they are quite active in finance and tax management. However, unlike the majority of their counterparts in America, they only infrequently get involved in the management of clinical areas.

Staffing Levels

An issue that is crucial for all managers is staffing, and at first glance it would appear that Japanese hospitals have a magic formula. After all, their staffing ratios are almost one-third those of American hospitals. However, there are two problems with this statistic. First, despite appearances, Japanese hospital staffing ratios *are* essentially similar to those in American hospitals. As already noted, hospitals in Japan offer a wider range of services than those in the United States. So how do we compare staffing ratios in Japan and the United States? My suggestion is to apply a staff to bed ratio (SBR). Basically, this statistic measures how many staff are needed per bed turnover each year. In a general way this addresses the question of intensity of care, since the greater the intensity, the higher the ratio will be. The statistic is computed as follows:

$$SBR = \frac{\text{number of bed turnovers per year}}{\text{total number of hospital staff}}$$

Where, number of bed turnovers per year =
365/average length of stay

Using such a statistic produces much more comparable figures between the United States and Japan. Even within Japan it is apparent that St. Luke's staffing ratio is double that of other comparable Japanese hospitals—but its average length of stay is only half that of these other hospitals. Thus the SBR is almost the same for St. Luke's and other Japanese hospitals. Clearly, more research is needed on this point.

A second staffing data issue is that to a significant extent, staffing is understated in Japanese hospitals. In many institutions, it is expected and planned that some minimal level of nursing care will be provided by the patient's family. Also, hospital patients frequently employ personal aides, yet these aides are not considered part of the official work force. Finally, private nurses may be employed at the request of the family if the hospital does not have what is called "standard nursing," for which the hospital receives extra reimbursement. In the absence of "standard nursing," 70 percent of the costs of private nurses are reimbursed to the family through the national health insurance plan.

JAPANESE STYLE MANAGEMENT IN JAPANESE HOSPITALS

Japanese hospitals exist within the culture of Japan, and there are many aspects of Japanese style management that function in these institutions, including permanent employment, recruitment and orientation techniques, team building techniques, work relationships, and finally, the organization's holistic approach to the employee.

Permanent Employment

Permanent employment is the term I choose to use, rather than the more popular "lifetime employment." It should be made clear that permanent employment, even in the largest of industrial firms, only spans a period from the time the employee enters the organization until retirement age, which is usually 55. A second limitation is that in the event of financial reverses employees can be temporarily laid off, often for long stretches. Other limitations include that permanent employment has not been extended to women, and it is not available in smaller organizations. However, in the hospitals I visited and studied, permanent employment was a reality for all full-time staff, including nurses, all of whom were women. Further, I did not find any hospital manager who could recall firing any employee in the last five or ten years. Returning to the concept of *amae*, one would no doubt conclude that the firing of a staff member would reflect more on the inadequacy of the Japanese manager than of the staff person who had been fired.

It should also be recognized that permanent employment has a clear value to both hospital management and labor. For managers, it means a stable work force and that every dollar of training invested in an employee will be used for the betterment of the organization. For labor, there is a reasonable guarantee of employment during difficult economic times, protection against inequitable treatment, and finally, the benefit of being able to personally invest in an organization. It would be spurious to contend that permanent employment makes all employees in the Japanese hospitals equals. Clearly, there are status differentials based on sex, occupation, and age. Yet, permanent employment does mean that when appropriate, the nurse can speak up, even challenge the physician, without the fear of reprisal so common in American hospitals.

Staff Recruitment

While there are some interesting and important differences in Japanese, as compared to American, methods of recruiting and orienting new staff, the Japanese do not have a magic formula. As in the United States, applicants for positions are obtained through advertisements, contacts with training institutions (such as nursing schools and colleges), and finally, personal networks. Hospitals do not have some secret screening device (such as a Japanese version of the Minnesota Multiphasic Personality Inventory) that works with astounding accuracy. Rather, like their counterparts in America, they use the age-old approach of application review, reference checking, and subjective-based interviewing.

However, in Japan there is one significant difference: the "recruiting season." The school year in Japan runs from April to March, and the recruiting season appears to be from September through March, with all new employees, virtually in every organization throughout the country, starting on April 1st. To job seekers, this provides the opportunity to see what is available in each organization they are interested in, and for the organization, it provides the opportunity to look over the entire range of job applicants.

Staff Orientation

The hiring of a new group of employees, all of whom begin working at the same time, is of particular importance because it allows hospitals to invest heavily in one orientation program. Unlike American hospitals, which frequently hire and start new employees either every day (250 starts per year) or every week (52 starts per year), the Japanese hospital has one employee starting date per year. The orientation programs observed in Japan ranged in time from three or four days to three weeks. It must be noted that these were the general hospital orientations, not the department orientations, such as nursing, which often lasted months. As described in the St. Luke's case, the orientation period is an effective vehicle for indoctrinating the new employee into the ethos of the hospital and beginning the process of building a broad-based hospital team. However, it did appear that physicians were not involved in the orientation programs. This, in my opinion, is a most unfortunate missed opportunity. Indeed, it simply reinforces the status differences and potential communication difficulties between physicians and other hospital staff.

Team Building

The orientation period then becomes the first of many steps in building a team attitude within the hospital. Virtually every institution has a variety of hospital-sponsored sports teams and extracurricular activities, such as hiking or ski clubs, flower arranging clubs, and so on. Perhaps what is most significant is that while the hospital pays for part of these activities, the employees contribute to a welfare fund to pay a share themselves. In addition to these obvious social activities, supervisors are expected to play an active role in developing a team attitude within their work group. For example, one case study describes a radiologist who periodically goes out for dinner and sake with his technicians and then, once or twice a year, takes an overnight trip with the staff. This is not unusual. At another level, and apparently in the private hospitals, periodic large meetings or song singing might take place. However, it should be emphasized that in the one private hospital presented in the cases, employees viewed monthly song singing as a somewhat pleasurable respite rather than a statement of loyalty to the hospital.

Finally, it should be recognized that this type of team building is most effective with the general duty employees and least effective with the doctors. In essence, the general duty employees must become integral parts of the team, since they have limited job mobility and few skills that are marketable outside of the organization. The nurses, to some degree, and the physicians, to the greatest extent, are relatively independent professionals who, in the tradition of all professionals, answer to a higher calling (and also have greater job mobility than the general duty employees).

Worker Relationships

Work and worker relationships are often cited as a particularly unique dimension of the Japanese work force. The common view is that to the Japanese worker, the job is life itself. To some degree this attitude is borne out in the hospital field. Nurses frequently live in hospital housing, and their lives revolve around the organization; their friends come from the hospital, and vacations are spent with hospital colleagues at hospital-owned resorts. Among men, such socialization occurs to an even greater degree, and as the survey indicated, the breakdown of social relationships within the hospital could result in problems for the Japanese worker.

Middle managers, such as department heads, frequently develop relationships with workers that continue after work hours. It must be assumed that this is a policy that the hospital either encourages or, at the least, does not discourage. The American (or perhaps western) view of familiarity breeding contempt apparently does not apply here. Indeed, the sense is quite the contrary: familiarity breeds loyalty.

Based on my visits to a number of administrative offices, it is apparent that this sense of familiarity is manifested even in the physical surroundings. In general, the offices had a well-lived-in atmosphere and were almost always large, open spaces, with many desks abutting one another. Typically, the staff person, usually a man and often referred to in Japan as a salaryman, came to work in a suit. Shortly after arriving he would remove his jacket and shoes, put on slippers and sweater, and go about his business. This scene, witnessed numerous times, was reminiscent of the opening scenes of Mr. Roger's Neighborhood, and interestingly enough, the offices had almost the same sense of warmth and family of one's own living room. The sterility and impersonality too often found in the American office simply did not exist. The message was hardly subtle—in your office you are home and among friends.

An interesting dimension of the work relationship relates to the role of women and is best illustrated with the following story. One morning I was observing the operations of the accounting and finance section of a hospital's business office. Eight people, seven men and one woman, worked in the office. With the exception of one supervisor and one new staff person, the others did the same type of accounting work. During the morning the group appeared to be working along in an amiable fashion, and the woman participated in most conversations. At noon the workers cleared their desks, and the woman went to the cafeteria to pick up the box lunches for all her male colleagues, delivered them to their desks, and then cleaned up when the meal was finished. Liberation, in the American sense, only goes so far in the Japanese hospital.

Consensual Decision Making

Consensual decision making also goes "only so far" in the Japanese hospital. While *ringi* systems do exist, they are in large measure a function of a centralized budgeting system and represent a way of documenting and keeping records of decisions. It is clear, from the case studies and other site visits, that the important planning and service decisions are in the hands of the top medical and administrative staff. The technical-level staff do not appear to play any more of a role in decision making in Japan than in America.

Clearly, there is a holistic concern for the employee within the Japanese hospital. The organization perceives itself as responsible for the employee's total well-being and, by extension, for the well-being of the employee's family. Hospitals provide housing (in one case, loans to purchase housing), medical benefits, subsidized vacations, and in some cases, extensive continuing education programs.

When an employee gets married, the employee's supervisor will normally make a speech at the wedding and give the employee a generous gift. It still frequently happens that a staff member will ask his or her supervisor for advice and counsel about a pending engagement or wedding. At the wedding the place of honor (next to the groom or bride) is traditionally reserved for the "matchmaker" or "go between" who, by custom, is the groom's work supervisor, not the parents of the couple.

THE MAGIC FORMULA

To this point, the magic formula of Japanese management has not been revealed, and with good reason: there is no magic formula. The Japanese system works well in Japan, but it is not perfect. The doctors are not terribly interested in the team, staff do not offer enough suggestions for hospital improvement, nurse turnover averages 20 percent (low by American standards; high by Japanese standards), and some suggest that productivity may in some cases be low.

Yet, with all these problems, the Japanese worker does not appear to be as alienated from the organization as the American worker. Clearly, the work force in the typical Japanese hospital is significantly more homogeneous ethnically, and in terms of socialization, than the work force in most American hospitals.

The conclusion must be that while there is no magic formula, the Japanese experience does suggest some important lessons. The next, and final, chapter suggests ways in which American hospitals can adopt and adapt from the Japanese experience.

An Agenda for A.
Hospital Manage.

Several times each month I receive a long-distance telephone call that sounds something like this: "I am the administrator of Happy 'Valley Hospital in Tsorisville. We are thinking of developing quality circles at our hospital, and I wanted to talk to you about the way the Japanese go about using quality circles in their hospitals."

"Why are you so interested?" I ask.

"Well, a few weeks ago I went to a seminar on quality circles in hospitals, and I was really impressed," the administrator responds.

At this point I ask what is usually perceived as an irrelevant question: "How much time do you spend on the orientation of new employees?" The answer is usually between two and four hours.

My conversation with the caller points up the fact that there are no easy answers to the problems of hospital administration in America. Unions, medical staffs, regulations and regulators, courts, patient demands, and finances have made the hospital administrator's job a very difficult one indeed. The days when hospital administrators almost universally spoke of their job as "fun" are over. The demand placed upon hospital administration often results in a search for a quick fix or easy solution to a problem. In my judgment, the quality circle approach falls into this category. You simply cannot develop a quality circle program without simultaneously developing a range of other activities that makes fundamental changes in the quality of equitable practices and worklife in the institution. It is well to recall here the earlier-cited example of a hospital that was quite interested in quality circles but simply did not communicate in a basic way with its employees (although it worried considerably over its communications with medical staff). It is suggested that patchwork solutions such as quality circles, while of some short run value, have no viability in the long run.

Before presenting the elements of my agenda, it is necessary that the reader understand two of my philosophical positions. First, my view of human nature is

129

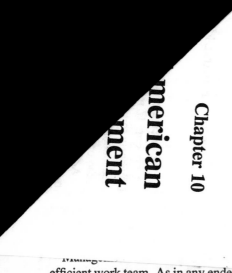

rustworthy, and not looking to rip off
...d accountable, they will respond.
...y have to be dealt with appropriately:
...al. In the Theory "X," Theory "Y"
...al Theory "Y" person.
...tive is my view that dissent, disagree-
...s of any search for the "best way."
...ment are often stifled or limited to an
...aff. Most of the staff are outside of the
...us, solutions usually appear imposed
...d, even if unworkable.
...to build a high-quality, effective, and
efficient work team. As in any endeavor, this cannot be done without a significant
investment in people by the organization. Simultaneously, the staff member must
be allowed to invest in the organization and see a return on that investment. But,
how is this done?

A FIVE-POINT AGENDA FOR CHANGE

Five significant organizational changes are proposed. Most of these changes at
first appear deceptively simple and straightforward, but if implemented as a
package they would have a profound impact on any organization, in particular, a
hospital, since this plan would change the traditional relationships among the
board, management, medical staff, and nonmedical staff. For example, under this
plan nurses or technicians would be enfranchised—they too would have a strong
voice in the future of the organization. No longer would the power differential
between the nursing staff and the medical staff be as acute as it is at present. The
changes enumerated on the following pages are organized under five headings:
(1) recruitment, (2) orientation, (3) permanent employment, (4) holism and
paternalism, and (5) communications.

Point 1—Recruitment

Hospitals should change their recruitment policies so that there is a recruitment
season. Typically, a 400-bed hospital with 1,400 employees might hire 500 new
people each year, with an average of 2 new hires each working day. This pattern of
hiring employees on an as-needed basis should be altered, so that new staff begin
working at the hospital no more than 12, and preferably only 4 times per year. If
new employees started once a month, then approximately 40 people would begin

Chapter 10

An Agenda for American Hospital Management

Several times each month I receive a long-distance telephone call that sounds something like this: "I am the administrator of Happy Valley Hospital in Tsorisville. We are thinking of developing quality circles at our hospital, and I wanted to talk to you about the way the Japanese go about using quality circles in their hospitals."

"Why are you so interested?" I ask.

"Well, a few weeks ago I went to a seminar on quality circles in hospitals, and I was really impressed," the administrator responds.

At this point I ask what is usually perceived as an irrelevant question: "How much time do you spend on the orientation of new employees?" The answer is usually between two and four hours.

My conversation with the caller points up the fact that there are no easy answers to the problems of hospital administration in America. Unions, medical staffs, regulations and regulators, courts, patient demands, and finances have made the hospital administrator's job a very difficult one indeed. The days when hospital administrators almost universally spoke of their job as "fun" are over. The demand placed upon hospital administration often results in a search for a quick fix or easy solution to a problem. In my judgment, the quality circle approach falls into this category. You simply cannot develop a quality circle program without simultaneously developing a range of other activities that makes fundamental changes in the quality of equitable practices and worklife in the institution. It is well to recall here the earlier-cited example of a hospital that was quite interested in quality circles but simply did not communicate in a basic way with its employees (although it worried considerably over its communications with medical staff). It is suggested that patchwork solutions such as quality circles, while of some short run value, have no viability in the long run.

Before presenting the elements of my agenda, it is necessary that the reader understand two of my philosophical positions. First, my view of human nature is that the vast majority of workers are honest, trustworthy, and not looking to rip off the system. If made responsible and held accountable, they will respond. Obviously some are loafers or worse, and they have to be dealt with appropriately: reeducation, redirection, and finally, removal. In the Theory "X," Theory "Y" dichotomy, I come down as a slightly cynical Theory "Y" person.

A second important philosophical perspective is my view that dissent, disagreement, and debate are essential components of any search for the "best way." However, in hospitals dissent and disagreement are often stifled or limited to an inner circle of administrators and medical staff. Most of the staff are outside of the consultative and decision processes, and thus, solutions usually appear imposed and are resisted or worse yet, implemented, even if unworkable.

Management's challenge, therefore, is to build a high-quality, effective, and efficient work team. As in any endeavor, this cannot be done without a significant investment in people by the organization. Simultaneously, the staff member must be allowed to invest in the organization and see a return on that investment. But, how is this done?

A FIVE-POINT AGENDA FOR CHANGE

Five significant organizational changes are proposed. Most of these changes at first appear deceptively simple and straightforward, but if implemented as a package they would have a profound impact on any organization, in particular, a hospital, since this plan would change the traditional relationships among the board, management, medical staff, and nonmedical staff. For example, under this plan nurses or technicians would be enfranchised—they too would have a strong voice in the future of the organization. No longer would the power differential between the nursing staff and the medical staff be as acute as it is at present. The changes enumerated on the following pages are organized under five headings: (1) recruitment, (2) orientation, (3) permanent employment, (4) holism and paternalism, and (5) communications.

Point 1—Recruitment

Hospitals should change their recruitment policies so that there is a recruitment season. Typically, a 400-bed hospital with 1,400 employees might hire 500 new people each year, with an average of 2 new hires each working day. This pattern of hiring employees on an as-needed basis should be altered, so that new staff begin working at the hospital no more than 12, and preferably only 4 times per year. If new employees started once a month, then approximately 40 people would begin each orientation period (even 24 starting periods would create a group of 20). Such a policy is an initial step in building cohesive work teams. Staff can begin to envision themselves as the class of '83, for example, or the group that started in the fall of '83. Generally speaking, the advertising, pool development, and interviewing of staff in American hospitals require few changes, although a continuing problem is that of obtaining accurate references.

Point 2—Orientation

The orientation period in American hospitals needs a drastic overhaul. The message sent to the employee, beginning on day 1, is that the hospital does not care about the new staff member and that the relationship will be a rather distant one. What is the message that is communicated during the four days at St. Luke's? I suggest it is a message of investment. The hospital is telling the employees that it cares about them and that they will play a significant role in the future of the organization. The presentations by the senior executives, the book discussion, the luncheons, the tour, and the final speaker create a sense of attachment rarely encountered in the American hospital.

When was the last time an American hospital included discussions on the hospital's history, its market position or marketing strategy, the long-range plan, or the role of the board in its new staff orientation? Better yet, what hospital has a board member participating in new employee orientation? When was the last time an orientation included a full-blown VIP tour of the hospital? A typical response to these inquiries is: "We don't have the time." The time must be found! Orientation is really socialization to the beliefs and values of the organization—its ethos and spirit. The message communicated during these first few days becomes etched deeper in the memory than any other message the employee is likely to receive over the next few years.

Obviously, if new staff begin 250 times a year, such an orientation program becomes exceedingly expensive and cumbersome. Starting new employees once a week, 52 times a year, makes developing the orientation program easier. (And of course, starting new employees twice a month (26 times a year), once a month (12 times per year), or once each quarter (4 times per year) makes it that much easier.)

Point 3—Permanent Employment

A crucial part of the agenda is rewarding core staff in every job category (perhaps 50 percent of the entire hospital staff) with permanent employment, contingent on the availability of funds (when certain conditions of satisfactory service and length of employment are met). In some American firms employees are given tenure after ten or fifteen years—in Japan, it happens after a several-month probationary period.

What does permanent employment do? First, it provides employees with job stability and thus allows them to make a return investment in the hospital. They know their future is dependent on the well-being of the institution and that after they have invested themselves, they will see a return on the investment. Second, it enfranchises within the hospital a group of persons who, until then, were essentially second-class citizens. Recently, an ICU nurse told me how she had been berated by a physician because she had suggested that a patient whose fever was rising rapidly (and not responding to drugs) be covered with a cooling blanket. The physician reminded the nurse that he had an M.D. after his name and that the nurse had an R.N. after hers, and that he was the only one around who gave orders. After this tirade he slammed the phone down, leaving a dumbstruck nurse and a very hot patient. This story is often repeated in one version or another throughout the health care system. Part of the problem is simply that there is no countervailing force to the doctor in the hospital. Permanent employment would, for the first time, set up that countervailing force; it would mean that the employees had a stake in what was happening and a powerful voice to express their viewpoint. Indeed, I would argue that if permanent employment existed, the need for unionization would dwindle, because hospitals would have taken a giant step forward toward the goal of becoming more democratic organizations.

Point 4—Holism and Paternalism

Two decades ago interns received a salary of $125.00 per month, plus room and board. The first level of competition for house staff was always on the basis of the quality of the medical education, but the second level of competition often revolved around housing. In one hospital where I worked, the salary was raised during the early 1960s to a "living wage" of $400.00 per month, but food privileges (first for the families and later, the house staff) were taken away. So, we thought, ends paternalism.

Many hospitals provide generous fringe benefits including medical care, pensions, subsidized meals, subsidized housing, and even theater tickets. But many of the benefits that are of particular importance to the typical salaried worker only find their way to the top-paid physicians. For example, I recall hearing the head of a medical department at a medical center tell me how he received several thousand dollars per year from the hospital for his daughter's tuition. At the time his salary was in excess of $100,000, and he could well afford to pay the tuition himself. But what about the nurse trying to send her teenager to college? Where was her tuition package?

There is no easy solution to the problem of demonstrating care and concern for the employee. However, the trend, primarily in industry, of offering the employee a smorgasbord of possible benefits and then helping him or her choose an appropriate package is certainly a step in the right direction. Setting up in-house counseling services for the alcoholic employee, day care centers for children of employees, and crisis counseling programs are also steps in the right direction. Perhaps the hospital could even pick up the older children of staff at local schools and provide them with a supervised after-school play program. Financial or technical assistance in securing mortgage loans should also be considered in the range of possible benefits. Career counseling services for employees and their families, in-service education, and tuition assistance are all programs that indicate a concern about the staff member's growth and development. Finally, the managers and middle managers must take the time, and the organization must support their efforts, to get to know their staff as people. Getting together for a relaxed lunch or supper will return psychic as well as organizational dividends; the annual Christmas party is simply not enough. Nor is it enough for these meals to go on during business hours or solely in the hospital cafeteria, where the manager's sense of territoriality is well protected.

Point 5—Communications

Many hospitals publish a weekly calendar of events. In order to save money they often distribute several copies to each department, one to each administrator, and one to each physician. What's the message? There are those who count, and those who don't count. While the interest in hospital marketing is a positive trend, I propose that more effort be expended on internal marketing. All staff members want and need to be kept informed. In several Japanese hospitals there is a 15-minute morning assembly where polite greetings are exchanged, followed by a report on the present status of the hospital, for example, occupancy, number of admissions and discharges, and any particularly noteworthy events. Everyone is told about the broken steam pipe and the herpes conference at three o'clock. In the typical American hospital, there is only the grapevine.

In one hospital where I worked, free coffee was served in the dining room from 10:00 A.M. to 11:00 A.M., and the custom was for the nursing staff, the administrators, and the entire medical staff to stop by during those hours. Informal communication worked well there, but a new administrator put a stop to that practice; he chose to save $80.00 a week instead. We need to examine our communications networks and plug in those who were never connected. It's hard to be a member of the team when you don't get the information.

We can all take a lesson from Detroit's Henry Ford Hospital, which places a "Newsbrief" card (which gives information on a daily basis about newsworthy items, including census data) on the center of each table in the staff dining room. It's an inexpensive and thoughtful way of keeping the staff informed.

PAYOFFS AND RISKS

Would following this agenda pay off in dollars? The direct payoff, it is proposed, would be in terms of reduced alienation, which should lead to a more efficient and effective work force.

A second measurable payoff should be reduced turnover and, hence, reduced personnel expenses for training and redevelopment. Additionally, it means that personnel development investments can be planned on a long-term basis.

But there are risks. The first risk relates to implementing the plan and then finding out that turnover has not decreased, production is the same, and alienation is just as high. Also, the hospital is stuck with a large number of permanent employees who act just like they always have. The social pressures that induce people to leave in Japan are not likely to have the same effect here. One response, as earlier suggested, might be to limit people and positions eligible for permanent employment. A second response might be to give it time. The importance and impact of most significant changes, getting married, having children, or obtaining tenure, for example, are not immediately obvious. If, after implementation and waiting, there is still no difference, the costs of the risks are probably not so high as to outweigh the second risk.

This second risk is that of doing nothing. Simply let the organization continue as it has for decades, absorbing the financial drain of alienated staff with high turnover and the emotional drain of a staff in turmoil.

It is suggested here that one of the few organizational levers most managers have to work with is staffing. Most choose to operate on a management-by-exception basis, but this leaves too much vital activity unmanaged. Managers must learn to anticipate problems and their solutions and to adapt the innovative ideas of their Japanese colleagues. In the long run the payoff will be for the staff, the patients, and the community.

Annotated Bibliography of Hospital Administration Books in Japanese

Compiled by Naoki Ikegami, M.D.

The following is an annotated bibliography of some of the major works in hospital and medical administration in Japan. The books are listed in alphabetical order, by author. All have been published in Tokyo.

H. Hashimoto and Y. Yoshida, editors
Comprehensive Handbook of Hospital Administration
Igaku Shoin, 1970–1980
Vol. 1 *History of Hospitals, Modern Hospitals, Medical Care System,*
Concept of Hospital Administration, Organization of Hospitals, Ethics (1972)
Vol. 2 *Practice of Hospital Administration,* Part I (1970)
Vol. 3 *Practice of Hospital Administration,* Part II (1971)
Vol. 4 *Hospital Management* (1970)
Vol. 5 *Hospital and Public Health* (1970)
Vol. 6 *Hospital Architecture, Hospital Equipment, and Medical Instruments,* Part I (1974);
Part II (1980)

This massive work, edited by the director of St. Luke's Hospital and by the director of the National Institute of Hospital Administration, can be considered as a cumulative conclusion of adapting MacEachern's *Hospital Organization and Management* into Japanese hospital administration. The authors include the leading persons in their respective fields and cover a wide range of subjects.

K. Ichijo
Analysis of Hospital Operation
Igaku Shoin, 1965; Revised Edition 1974

This book is based on the author's personal experience of analyzing over 200 hospitals. The major weight is given to productivity analyses, calculated from the financial ratio of each department. Clinical departments are also covered.

E. Imamura
Theory and Practice of Hospital Administration
Igaku Shoin, 1968

This volume outlines the history, function, and organization of hospitals; hospital ethics; and the structure of and relationship between medical departments. The importance of human relations and public relations to the hospital is noted.

S. Ishihara
Method and Examples of Hospital Management Analysis
Igaku Shoin, 1962

Case studies of hospitals, personally conducted by the author. Hospitals studied are mainly of the local government-owned type.

M. Kurata, editor
Techniques of Scientific Hospital Management
Igaku Shoin, 1964

The methodology of work simplification, human engineering, system engineering, stock administration, cost evaluation, etc., are explained, with their tentative application into hospitals.

M. Kurata
Hospital Planning
Kanehara Shuppan, 1970

This is the first book on hospital planning from the viewpoint of administrative medicine. The steps are shown to be defining the planning area, the role of the hospital, and planning the hospital's function.

M. Kurata and Y. Hayashi
Regional Health Planning
Shinohara Shuppan, 1977

The authors develop the theme described in *Hospital Planning*. The history of health planning is compared, in Japan and the United States. The concept of the planning area is outlined. Hayashi contributes in the areas of system engineering and information science.

T. Shimauchi
Hospital and Medical Care Administration
Igaku Shoin, First Ed. 1956; Second Ed. 1967

This work is in two parts: Part I is administrative medicine and concerns medical care as a system. Part II is hospital administration proper. This is the first work in Japanese providing a comprehensive outline of this new field and is based on the lectures the author gave at the Tohoku University Medical School.

M. Takahashi
Hospital Administration—An Introductory Manual
Igaku Shoin, First Ed. 1967; Second Ed. 1973

This is a short guide to the general concepts of hospital administration. The chapters include organization theory, human relations, ethics, divisional management, finance, and medical evaluation.

M. Yamamoto
Hospital Accounting, Theory, and Practice
Kanehara Shoten Edition 1944; Igaku Shoin First Ed. 1950, Second Ed. 1960, Third Ed. 1967

This pioneering work on hospital accounting is based almost entirely on the author's personal struggle to develop an accounting system for hospitals.

M. Yamamoto
Synopsis of Modern Hospital Management
Shinohara Shuppan, First Ed. 1977; Second Ed. 1980

The book is divided into sections on organizational theory, personnel management, and finance management. It is a cumulation of the author's lifetime work in hospital administration.

Selected English-Language Readings on Health Care in Japan

Broida, J.H. "Case Study of Physicians' Practice in Ambulatory Medical Care Setting—Japan," *Social Science and Medicine* 12 (1978): 555–561.

Broida, J.H., & Maeda, N. "Japan's High-Cost Illness Insurance Program, A Study of its First Three Years, 1974–1976." *Public Health Reports* 93, no. 2 (March–April, 1978): 153–160.

Caudill, W. "The Cultural and Interpersonal Context of Everyday Health and Illness in Japan and America," in *Asian Medical Systems*, ed. Charles Leslie (Berkeley: University of California Press, 1976), pp. 159–177.

Hashimoto, M. "A Case Study on Health Planning Methods in Japan—Comprehensive Community Health Planning," *Bulletin of the Institute of Public Health* 26, no. 3.4 (Tokyo: 1977): 125–141.

Hashimoto, M. "Health Care and Medical Systems in Japan," *Bulletin of the Institute of Public Health* 27, no. 1 (Tokyo: 1978): 1–18.

Hashimoto, S., & Kiikuni, K. *Health Services in Japan*, published for the 20th International Hospital Congress (Tokyo: 1977).

Ikegami, N. "Growth of Psychiatric Beds in Japan," *Social Science and Medicine* 14A (1980): 561–570.

Ikegami, N. "Institutionalized and the Non-Institutionalized Elderly," *Social Science and Medicine* 16 (1982): 2001–2008.

Iwasa, K. "Hospitals in Japan: History and Present Situation," *Medical Care* 4 (October–December, 1966): 241–246.

Japan Hospital Association, *Japan Hospital*, Serial Number 1 (July 1982).

S. Jonas, "Japan Struggles Under Complex Health System," *Hospitals* 49 (September 1975): 56–60.

Lock, M.M. *East Asian Medicine in Japan: Varieties of Medical Experience* (Berkeley: University of California Press, 1980).

Reich, R., & Kao, J., ed. *A Comparative View of Health and Medicine in Japan and America* (New York: Japan Society Inc., 1978).

Steslicke, W.E. *Doctors in Politics: The Political Life of the Japan Medical Association* (New York: Praeger, 1973).

Steslicke, W.E. "Development of Health Insurance Policy in Japan," *Journal of Health Politics, Policy and Law* 7, no. 1 (Spring 1982): 197–226.

Steslicke, W.E. "National Health Policy in Japan: From the Age of Flow to the Age of Stocks," *Bulletin of the Institute of Public Health* 31, no. 1 (1982): 1–35.

Yoshitake, Y. *Hospital Visits in Japan*, prepared by the Working Committee on Hospital Architecture for the 20th International Hospital Congress (Tokyo: 1977).

Index

A

Access, 4
Acute care institution concept, 119
Administration, 7-8
  attitudes toward, 111-112
  avoidance of decision making by, 8
  in Japan, 121, 122
  Japanese books on, 135-137
  nursing, 51-52
  personnel. *See* Personnel
    management
  physicians in, 37, 38
  training for, 38-39
  unit-level nursing, 51-52
Age
  differences in between U.S. and
    Japanese hospitals, 92-93
  mandatory retirement, 20-21
  and population base, 34-35
Alienation of workers, 6, 134
Amae, 19
American hospitals
  age differences between Japanese
    hospitals and, 92-93
  management of, 129-134
  permanent employment in, 131-132
American worker attitudes, 85-115
  vs. Japanese workers, 17
  towards selection of workplace,
    95-97

Analysis of Hospital Operation, 135
Anatomy of Dependence, The, 19
Attitudes
  toward administration, 111-112
  of American workers. *See*
    American worker attitudes
  of Japanese workers, 17, 94-95
  job leaving, 100-111
  mental, 16
  moral, 16
  toward supervision, 112-113
Average length of stay, 38

B

Benefits, 96, 97, 98, 108, 113, 132
Bonus awards at St. Luke's, 79
Books on hospital administration in
  Japanese, 135-137
Bottom-up initiative vs. top-down
  direction, 18
Broida, J.H., 139
Budget
  at Kitashinagawa Hospital, 61
  operating, 69
Businesses in Japan, 12
Business management in Japanese
  hospitals, 55-56

C

Caudill, W., 139
Central Social Insurance Medical
    Council, 31
CEO. *See* Chief executive officers
Chain of command, 22
Change in disease patterns, 4
Chapter 372 in Massachusetts, 4
Chief executive officers (CEO), 7
Chi-square analysis, 97-99
Climate of management, 101-104
Clinics, 120-121
Cole, R., 13
Command chain, 22
Communications, 133-134
    staff, 80-81
Company housing, 16
Company-oriented generalist
    managers, 11
*Comparative View of Health and
    Medicine in Japan and America, A,*
    139
*Comprehensive Handbook of Hospital
    Administration,* 135
Confined management development,
    21
Consensus decision making (ringi-
    seido), 11, 18, 127
Continuing education at St. Luke's,
    71-72, 76
Corporate stability, 22
Corporations in Japan, 20-21
Costs
    health care, 3-4
    medical technology, 34
    physician involvement in, 5
Coworker relationships, 21-22,
    100-101, 126-127
Cross-cultural studies, 86

D

Debate, 130
Decision making, 5

administrator avoidance of, 8
consensus, 11, 18, 127
medical staff in, 5
nurses in, 6
physicians in, 5
Deficit reduction at Public
    Corporation Hospital, 58
Delivery of health care, 34
Demography, 4
Diagnostic related grouping (DRG), 4
Direction, 18
Disadvantages of Japanese system, 20
Disagreement, 130
Disease pattern changes, 4
Dissent, 130
*Doctors in Politics: The Political Life
    of the Japan Medical Association,*
    139
Doi, Takeo, 19
DRG. *See* Diagnostic related grouping
Drucker, Peter, F., 7, 15, 21

E

*East Asian Medicine in Japan:
    Varieties of Medical Experience,*
    139
Economic conditions, 107-109
Education
    continuing, 71-72, 76
    manager, 21-22
    nursing, 82-83
Employees
    See also Personnel management;
        Staff
    evaluation of at St. Luke's, 77
    female, 16
    holistic concern for, 11, 16-17,
        127, 132-133
    lifetime. *See* Permanent employment
    new, 129
    permanent. *See* Permanent
        employment
    potential, 16

social programs for, 16
temporary, 15, 16
England, 121
English-language readings on health
  care in Japan, 139-140
Enterprise unions, 13-14
Episcopal Medical Mission, 67-68
Equitable access, 4
Escalator approach, 20
Ethical issue of equitable access, 4
Ethnically homogeneous work force
  in Japan, 14-15
Evaluation, 20
  informal, 21
  at Public Corporation Hospital, 50
  at St. Luke's, 73, 77
Expenses at St. Luke's, 70

F

Factory worker attitudes, 17
Federal government, 4
Fee variation, 33
Female employees in Japan, 16
Finance of St. Luke's 69-70
Fringe benefits, 96, 97, 98, 108,
  113, 132

G

GAO. *See* General Accounting Office
General Accounting Office (GAO), 5
General hospital concept, 119
Generalists, 57-58
  company-oriented, 11
  vs. specialists, 18-19
Gibney, F., 18, 19
Goldsmith, Seth B., 27
Governments, 4
Group identity vs. professional
  identity, 20

H

Hanami, Tadashi, 15
Hashimoto, H., 135
Hashimoto, M., 139
Hashimoto, S., 139
Hayashi, Y., 136
Health care
  costs of, 3-4, 5
  delivery of, 34
  English-language readings on in
    Japan, 139-140
  in Japan, 28, 139-140
  long-term, 119
  physician involvement in costs of, 5
  planning of delivery of, 34
  westernization influences on in
    Japan, 28
Health insurance
  in Japan, 29-33
  national, 121-122
Health status indices, 35
  in Japan, 27
Henry Ford Hospital, Detroit, 133
Hiring at St. Luke's, 76-77
History
  of Japan, 27-29
  of St. Luke's, 67-68
Holism, 11, 16-17, 127, 132-133
*Hospital Accounting, Theory, and
  Practice*, 137
*Hospital Administration - An
  Introductory Manual*, 137
Hospital board power, 7
*Hospital and Medical Care
  Administration*, 136
Hospital Planning, 136
Hospital Visits in Japan, 140
Housing, 16

I

Ichijo, K., 135
Identity, 20
Ikegami, Naoki, 27, 139

Imamura, E., 136
Income. *See* Revenue
Industry in Japan, 12, 13
Inflation, 4
Informal evaluations, 21
Information management at
  Kitashinagawa Hospital, 62
In-house training at Public
  Corporation Hospital, 50
Initiative, 18
Insurance, 29-33, 121-122
Interdependency, 19
Investments
  in nursing education, St. Luke's,
    82-83
  personnel development, 134
Ishihara, S., 136
Iwasa, K., 139

J

Japan
  attitudes of factory workes, in, 17
  disadvantages of system in, 20
  English-language readings on health
    care in, 139-140
  ethnically homogeneous work force
    in, 14-15
  female employees in, 16
  health insurance system in, 29-33
  health service in, 27-36
  health status indices in, 27
  history of, 27-29
  hospital administration books on,
    135-137
  hospital management in, 37-44
  hospital workers' attitudes and
    opinions in, 85-115
  implications of system in, 21-22
  "magic formula" of management
    in, 128
  managerial success in, 11, 15-19
  Medical Services Law of, 37, 122
  National Institute of Hospital
    Administration in, 39, 86

rising through corporations in,
  20-21
size of industry in, 12, 13
small businesses in, 12
unionization in, 13-14
westernization influences on health
  care in, 28
worker attitudes towards selection
  of workplace in, 94-95
Japanese hospitals
  administrators in, 121, 122
  age differences between U.S.
    hospitals and, 92-93
  business managers in, 122
  long-term care role in, 119
  management of, 122-123, 124-127
  staffing levels in, 123
  staff orientation in, 125
  staff recruitment in, 124-125
  team building in, 125-126
  worker relationships in, 126-127
Japanese Red Cross Medical Center,
  42-43
"Japan, Inc.," 12-13
Job leaving attitudes, 100-111
Job shifting, 20
Jonas, S., 139

K

Kao, J., 139
Keio University School of Medicine,
  38, 39
Kiikuni, K., 139
Kitashinagawa Hospital, 59-66, 85
  attitudes of employees at, 103, 104,
    109, 110, 113
  attitudes toward supervision at, 113
  budget at, 61
  coworker relationships at, 101
  and hospital quality, 109, 110
  information management at, 62
  job leaving attitudes at, 103
  managerial organization at, 62
  managerial philosophy at, 62-63

nursing department at, 64
patient volume at, 61
personnel manager at, 64-65
radiology department at, 63-64
staffing at, 61, 65-66
Kohno Clinical Medicine Research
  Institute, 59
Kohno, Minoru, 59-60, 63, 64-65, 66
Kurata, M., 136

L

Labor unions. *See* Unions
Length of stay, 119
  average, 38
Lifetime employment. *See* Permanent
  employment
Lock, M.M., 139
Long-range planning, 22
Long-run orientation, 11
Long-term care role in Japanese
  hospitals, 119
Loyalty of staff at Public Corporation
  Hospital, 56-57
Lump sum payment (taishokukin) at
  St. Luke's, 79

M

MacEachern, *, 39
Maeda, N., 139
"Magic formula" of Japanese
  management, 128
Malpractice suits, 34
Managerial generalists at Public
  Corporation Hospital, 57-58
Managerial philosophy at
  Kitashinagawa Hospital, 62-63
Manager rotation, 19, 20, 49
Mandatory retirement age, 20-21
Massachusetts Chapter, 372, #4
Medical vs. nonmedical management
  practices at Public Corporation
  Hospital, 56

Medical Services Law of Japan, 37,
  122
Medical staff
  See also Physicians
  in decision making, 5
  organization of, 120-121
Medical technology, 4
  cost of, 34
Mental attitudes, 16
Mentors, 21
*Method and Examples of Hosptial
  Management Analysis,* 136
Middle management, 126
  rotation of at Public Corporation
    Hospital, 49
Minnesota Multiphasic Personality
  Inventory, 125
Misconduct of physicians, 8
Moral attitudes, 16
Mutual interdependency, 19

N

Nakane, Chie, 16
National health insurance, 121-122
National Health Survey, 32
National Institute of Hospital
  Administration, Japan, 39, 86
National Medical Center, 41-42
Negotiations with unions, 77-78
New-employee orientation. *See*
  Orientation
"Newsbrief" card, 133
Nippon Recruit Center, 16
Nonmedical vs. medical management
  practices at Public Corporation
  Hospital, 56
Northwestern University, 39
Number of hospitals, 37
Nursing
  and decision making, 6
  education in at St. Luke's, 82-83
  at Kitashinagawa Hospital, 64
  at Public Corporation Hospital,
    51-54

relationship between physicians and
  at Public Corporation Hospital,
  54
shortages in, 5
"standard," 123
at St. Luke's, 70-75, 71
unit-level administration of, 51-52
Nursing homes, 119

O

Operating budget at St. Luke's, 69
Opportunities, 96, 97, 99
Organization
  of management at Kitashinagawa
    Hospital, 62
  of medical staff, 120-121
  of nursing department at St.
    Luke's, 71
  of St. Luke's, 68-69, 71
Organizational orientation toward
  long run, 11
Organization chart at St. Luke's, 68
Orientation, 16, 17, 129
  in Japanese hospitals, 125
  long-run, 11
  at St. Luke's, 80, 125
Outpatient clinics, 120-121
Ownership of hospitals, 37
  private, 121

P

Paternalism, 132-133
Patient volume, 32-33
  at Kitashinagawa Hospital, 61
Pay scale, 96, 97, 98
  at Public Corporation Hospital,
    50-51
  at St. Luke's, 78-79
Pediatrics ward at St. Luke's, 73-75
Pension system at St. Luke's, 79
Permanent employment, 11, 15, 16,
  124
  in American hospitals, 131-132

Personnel management
  See also Employees; Staff
  at Kitashinagawa Hospital, 64-65
  nursing, 52-53
  at Public Corporation Hospital,
    48-51
  at St. Luke's 76-81
Philosophy of management at
  Kitashinagawa Hospital, 62-63
Physicians
  See also Medical staff
  and decision making, 5
  and health care costs, 5
  as hospital administrators, 37, 38
  misconduct of, 8
  power of, 6, 7
  relationship between nurses and at
    Public Corporation Hospital, 54
Planning
  of health care delivery, 34
  long-range, 22
Point-fee system, 29-31
Population base aging, 34-35
Potential employees, 16
Power
  of hospital boards, 7
  of physicians, 6, 7
Primary care practitioner function,
  121
Private ownership of hospitals, 121
Productivity, 6, 128
Professional identity vs. group
  identity, 20
Professional opportunities, 96, 97, 99
Professional societies, 28
Professional unionization, 6
Promotions, 11, 20
Public Corporation Hospital, 47-58,
  85
  ages at, 92
  attitudes of employees at, 94, 100,
    101, 103, 109-110
  business management at, 55-56
  deficit reduction at, 58
  and hospital quality, 109-110

in-house training at, 50
job leaving attitudes at, 100, 101,
103
managerial generalists at, 57-58
medical vs. nonmedical management
practices at, 56
middle management rotation at, 49
nursing department at, 51-54
nursing personnel management at,
52-53
personnel administration at, 48-51
52-53
physician-nurse relationships at, 54
radiology department at, 54-55
staff evaluation at, 50
staff loyalty at, 56-57
staff pay scale at, 50-51
supervisory functions at, 52
team spirit at, 53
training programs at, 52
turnover at, 49
union membership at, 53
unit-level nursing administration at,
51-52
work group stratification at, 57
workplace selection attitudes at, 94

Q

Quality circles, 13, 41, 129
Quality of hospitals, 109-111

R

Racism, 12
Radiology department
at Kitashinagawa Hospital, 63-64
at Public Corporation Hospital,
54-55
at St. Luke's 75-76
Recruitment, 130-131
in Japanese hospitals, 124-125
at St. Luke's, 72-73, 76-77

Red Cross Medical Center in Japan,
42-43
Regional Health Planning, 136
Reich, R., 139
Relationships
coworker, 21-22, 100-101, 126-127
physician-nurse, at Public
Corporation Hospital, 54
with superiors, 22
supervisory, 104-106, 113
Relocation, 20
Retention at St. Luke's, 72-73
Retirement age, 20-21
Revenue
increase of, 31-32
at St. Luke's, 69-70
Ringi-seido (consensus decision
making), 11, 18, 127
Rotation of managers, 19, 20, 49

S

Salary structure. *See* Pay scale
Sasaki, N., 21
SBR. *See* Staff to bed ratio
Shimauchi, T., 136
"Shinryo," 62
Shortages of nurses, 5
Size
of hospitals, 37
of Japanese industry, 12, 13
Small businesses in Japan, 12
Social Insurance Medical Care Fee
Payment Fund, 31
Social programs for employees, 16
Sophia University, 15
Specialist vs. generalist approach,
18-19
Stability of corporations, 22
Staff
See also Employees; Personnel
management
development investments in, 134
at Kitashinagawa Hospital, 61,
65-66

levels of in Japanese hospitals, 123
loyalty at, 56-57
management of. *See* Personnel
management
medical. *See* Medical staff;
Physicians
orientation of. *See* Orientation
of outpatient clinics, 120-121
problems with, 5-6
productivity of, 6, 128
recruitment of. *See* Recruitment
survey of, 88-92
turnover in. *See* Turnover
Staff to bed ratio (SBR), 123
"Standard nursing," 123
State governments, 4
Stay length, 119
average, 38
Stereotyping of Japanese industry, 12
Steslicke, W.E., 139, 140
St. Luke's International Hospital,
Tokyo, 67-83
ages at, 92
attitudes of employees at, 94, 96,
109, 110, 112, 113
attitudes toward administration at,
112
attitudes toward supervision at, 113
bonus awards at, 79
continuing education at, 71-72, 76
coworker relationships at, 101
expenses of, 70
finance of, 69-70
hiring at, 76-77
history of, 67-68
and hospital quality, 109
investment in nursing education at,
82-83
job leaving attitudes at, 109, 110
location of, 96
loyalty at, 94
lump sum payment (taishokukin) at,
79
nursing at, 70-75
nursing department organization at,
71

operating budget of, 69
organization of, 68-69
orientation at, 80, 125
pediatrics ward at, 73-75
pension system at, 79
personnel evaluations at, 77
personnel management at, 76-81
radiology department at, 75-76
recruitment at, 72-73, 76-77
retention at, 72-73
revenue of, 69-70
salary structure at, 78-79
staff communication at, 80-81
staff evaluation at, 73
staffing ratio at, 123
turnover at, 72
union negotiation at, 77-78
Stratification of work group at Public
Corporation Hospital, 57
Success of Japanese management, 11,
15-19
Supervision, 112-113
Supervisory functions at Public
Corporation Hospital, 52
Supervisory relationships, 104-106,
113
Survey of hospital staff, 88-92
*Synopsis of Modern Hospital
Management*, 137

T

Taishokukin (lump sum payment) at
St. Luke's, 79
Takahashi, M., 137
Takezawa, S., 17
Teaching hospitals, 28
Teams, 130
in Japanese hospitals, 125-126
at Public Corporation Hospital, 53
*Techniques of Scientific Hospital
Management*, 136
Technology, 4
cost of, 34
Temporary employees, 15, 16

Teusler, Rudolf, 67, 68
Theory and Practice of Hospital Administration, 136
Theory "X," Theory "Y," 130
Toffler, A., 12
Toffler, H., 12
Tokuda, Torao, 43, 44
Tokushu-Kai Medical Corporation, 43-44
Tokyo Private Corporation Hospital, 40-41
Top-down direction vs. bottom-up initiative, 18
Toyota, 21
Training
hospital administration, 38-39
management, 21-22
at Public Corporation Hospital, 50, 52
Turnover, 6, 22, 134
at Public Corporation Hospital, 49
at St. Luke's, 72

professional, 6
at Public Corporation Hospital, 53
at St. Luke's, 77-78
United States. *See* American
Unit-level nursing administration at Public Corporation Hospital, 51-52
U.S. *See* American

W

Westernization influences on health care in Japan, 28
Whitehill, A., 17
Witt Associates, 7
Worker alienation, 6, 134
Worker orientation. *See* Orientation
Work group stratification at Public Corporation Hospital, 57
Workplace selection, 93-97
Work stoppages, 23
Woronoff, J., 13

U

Unions, 6
enterprise, 13-14
in Japan, 13-14

Y

Yamamoto, M., 137
Yoshida, Y., 135
Yoshitake, Y., 140

About the Author

SETH B. GOLDSMITH is a professor of public health in the health administration program at the University of Massachusetts at Amherst. Formerly chairman of the program and before that director of the graduate program in health services administration at the Columbia University School of Public Health, he has also served as a full-time faculty member of Tulane University and the Naval School of Hospital Administration. Dr. Goldsmith received his undergraduate degree in 1961 from New York University, where he majored in industrial and labor relations; his master's degree from the hospital administration program at Columbia University in 1963; and his doctorate from Johns Hopkins University in 1970. He has consulted with numerous hospitals, governmental agencies, and private organizations. He is editor of the *Journal of Ambulatory Care Management* and author of five books including *Ambulatory Care,* published by Aspen Systems in 1977. He is also author of *Health Care Management* (Aspen, 1981), a volume that was awarded a Book of the Year Award by the American Journal of Nursing in 1982.